JUN - 8 2019

D0456925

GENE EATING

GENE EATING

THE SCIENCE OF OBESITY
AND THE TRUTH ABOUT DIETING

GILES YEO, PhD

PEGASUS BOOKS
NEW YORK LONDON

GENE EATING

Pegasus Books, Ltd.
148 West 37th Street, 13th Floor
New York, NY 10018

Copyright © 2019 by Giles Yeo, PhD

First Pegasus Books hardcover edition June 2019

All rights reserved. No part of this book may be reproduced in whole
or in part without written permission from the publisher, except by reviewers
who may quote brief excerpts in connection with a review in a newspaper, magazine,
or electronic publication; nor may any part of this book be reproduced, stored in a
retrieval system, or transmitted in any form or by any means electronic, mechanical,
photocopying, recording, or other, without written permission from the publisher.

ISBN: 978-1-64313-127-6

10 9 8 7 6 5 4 3 2 1

For Jane

CONTENTS

PART 4 PROBLEM OF OUR TIME

INTRODUCTION

It was the first day of filming for the BBC Horizon's *Clean Eating* programme – a documentary investigating the 'dirty' truth behind pseudoscience fad diets – and we were heading into the hills north of San Diego to meet with Dr Robert O. Young, father of the 'alkaline diet'. I signalled left and moved smoothly into the fast lane on Interstate 15, as I headed north out of San Diego on a warm September morning. Normally, the rental vehicles utilised by the BBC are, well, rental-like; functional 'people mover' caravan-type things, which allow for the crew and all of their associated gear to be jammed in the back. On this sun-kissed Californian day, however, I was driving a silver Ford Mustang convertible, with the top down. The ridiculously large engine growled in response to the slightest squeeze of my right foot on the accelerator, while the wind blew through my hair . . . or at least it would have if I had any hair. I was living the dream!

Just over an hour later, I drove through some groves of avocado trees, and entered a millionaire's paradise that has become known as the 'pH Miracle Ranch'. Robert's 'pH Miracle' series of books have sold more than four million copies, and this beautifully manicured ranch is the epicentre of his multi-million dollar 'alkaline' empire. I manoeuvred the Mustang through the open gates of the white stone entrance down the long drive, and was soon joined by the crew, who had been following along behind in a far more sedate and 'rental-like' Dodge Caravan.

The front door, preposterously set behind a moat, is reached by walking across some stone slabs. As Robert welcomed me in, crew in tow with cameras rolling, my eyes were drawn to an empty spherical fish-tank built into the wall that separated the living area from the kitchen. Noting my interest, Robert began to share his alkaline view of the world, starting with what he called the fish bowl metaphor.

'If the fish is sick – what would you do? Treat the fish or change the water?'

He went on: 'The human body in its perfect state of health is alkaline in its design.'

Like many of the fad diets that are currently *en vogue*, this one begins with a kernel of truth. The pH of our blood is 7.4, which is slightly alkaline, so Robert is broadly correct; although different compartments of our bodies, such as our stomach, function at very different pHs. Everything else about 'alkaline living' however, is complete fantasy. Robert believes that in order to maintain the alkaline pH of our blood, we have to eat alkaline foods. The problem is, there is NO evidence that your blood's pH is influenced by what you eat. Your stomach, at around pH 1.5 (stronger than lemon juice or vinegar), is the most acidic environment in your body. So whatever you eat will arrive in your intestine at the same acidic pH. In fact, nothing apart from almost dying will change your blood's pH.

Why has the alkaline phenomenon exploded, if the (pseudo) science behind it doesn't even stand up to casual scrutiny? For that matter, why do people buy into 'clean'-eating, or 'plant-based', or detox, or juice cleansing, diets?

GETTING LUNCH? IT'S A JUNGLE OUT THERE!

Has there ever been a time in history where there have been so many dietary options? I mean, there is gluten-free, dairy-free, fat-free, nut-free, egg-free, sugar-free, shellfish-free ... the list goes on. I was lining up for coffee the other morning and the lady in front of me asked for a 'grande soy-decaf-latte with a shot of sugar-free caramel'. (Say that quickly three times in a row after you've had a few too many.)

A few years ago, for the first time, I saw a festive advertisement campaign from a major supermarket chain inviting potential customers to 'Have your "Free-From" Christmas celebrations with us!' Now, call me a cynic, but I do not think that the 'Free-From' festive ad campaign was solely aimed at the 1 per cent of the population that suffer from coeliac disease (who are allergic to gluten and therefore have to stay away from it). Nor do I, for one moment, imagine that the proliferation of non-dairy substitutes, such as soy, oat or almond milks, by major coffee purveyors is part of a drive to attract more lactose-intolerant customers (such as myself, although my preferred poison, not by chance, is a black Americano). Nope, these 'Free-From' foods are being marketed as more 'healthy'.

The term 'healthy' is, I would argue, in the eye of the beholder. If you have a broken leg, you want your leg to heal. If you have heart disease or cancer, well then, 'healthy' would mean to rid yourself of disease. And for many overweight and obese people out there, being 'healthy' would mean to lose weight.

Our modern lifestyle, coupled with the food environment, has made obesity the biggest public health problem of today, with up to 30 per cent of people in many countries carrying way too much fat. Aside from occasionally moonlighting as a science presenter for the BBC, I am first and foremost a scientist at the University of Cambridge, studying the control of bodyweight. I am an obesity geneticist. I, and many others, have spent the last two decades trying to understand what is perceived by most people on the planet as quite a simple problem. This is, by far and away, the prevailing view, and it is easy to see why. People just have to eat less and move more and they will lose weight. It is one of the fundamental laws of physics; you cannot magic calories out of nowhere, and likewise you cannot magic weight away.

The question to ask, however, is not how we have become obese (we do eat too much and move too little), but WHY some people eat more than others. The answer to this question is hugely complex, and we are only now beginning to reveal and understand the powerful genetic and biological influences on food intake. In doing so, other salient questions have emerged. Why do some people put on weight easily while others can apparently 'eat whatever they want'? How come some folks find it harder to lose weight than others? Why is the battle to maintain a 'healthy' weight so difficult for so many? The fact of the matter is that while simplistic 'eat-less' advice will work for some, for most of us, losing weight and then trying to keep it off is incredibly difficult. It is not what we are evolved to do, and the reality is, while we are making progress in understanding the problem, an all-encompassing solution remains out of reach. In this book, I will place the obesity epidemic in perspective, by explaining our current understanding of how food intake is controlled, how this differs between people, and how our genes influence our interaction with the environment. Science is set-up to get to the truth . . . eventually. It is not designed to provide quick answers. So here we are with an enormous contemporary problem of obesity and other diet-related illnesses, and a complete lack of quick and easy answers. As a result, there are many desperate people looking for a way out, a silver bullet.

EAT LIKE THIS AND LOOK LIKE ME

In response to this demand, a proliferation of food 'gurus' have in recent years emerged to fill the vacuum that nature so abhors, armed with confidently certain and easy-to-follow dietary approaches. If you spend any period of time exploring this, often social-media-dominated, world, you'll notice the reek of 'post-truth' that permeates the entire culture. It is clear that many are more likely to believe the advice of these food gurus than listen to experts who are taking an evidence-based approach to nutrition. In truth, we scientists don't always help the situation either, by having closed conversations in ivory research towers. What I hope to do in this book is to address that balance.

Supporters of eating 'clean' or 'real' food argue that it means enjoying whole foods in their most natural state, and limiting anything processed, which, on the face of it, seems to make sense. Who am I to argue with less refined sugar, less fast-food and more veggies? I am the first to agree that in this era of industrialised food production, in a drive for ever-greater efficiencies to create more for less, we have somehow broken our food environment. It is an environment we are going to have to fix in order to have a fighting chance to solve the obesity epidemic.

I do however, have major problems with these most modern of diet phenomena. First and foremost is the use of the word 'clean' or 'real'. Because if some foods are labelled clean or real, then the rest must, by definition, be 'dirty' or 'false' to some degree. Hence, through guilt by association with our diet, some of us could be considered 'clean' and others 'dirty'. I could be 'real' and you could be 'false'. This kind of 'food-shaming' is enormously unhealthy. It is my hope that this book will make society rethink its sweeping and negative judgements about obese people. Second, 'clean' and 'real' have, over the past few years, morphed into meaning 'food is medicine', and under this umbrella now includes a number of strains of diets, some more whacky than others, but all based on a foundation of pseudoscience.

SCIENCE-FICTION OR NON-FICTION?

I approach this book from the perspective of a geneticist with more than twenty years of experience studying obesity and the brain control of food intake. I was in the initial vanguard that described a number of genes that, when mutated, resulted in rare forms of severe obesity, thus uncovering key pathways in the brain that control food intake. My current research focusses on understanding how these pathways differ between lean and obese people, and the influence of genes in our feeding behaviour. However, I realise that in order to effectively tackle the problem of obesity, we also need to understand our food environment. I believe that this includes holding to account the exponential growth of dietary approaches and solutions that are being sold to us, and I spend a large part of this book doing just that. Just so we're crystal clear, this is NOT a diet book. It contains no diet-plan designed to make people lose weight and me lots of money. This is, in fact, an **Anti-'Diet' book**. Consider it a structured diatribe against dietary misinformation backed by bad (or no) science.

In this book, I will get to the truth and in doing so demystify the myriad of different popular dietary approaches available today. I will deconstruct the concept of a calorie and take a closer look at our obsession with counting these small units of energy. I will examine the truths and fallacies in the claims made by the Palaeolithic and 'clean' movements, while charting the actual history of our diet as we transitioned from stone-age hunter gatherers to farmers during the agricultural revolution, to the industrialised food production of today. I will explore the science-fiction and non-fiction of current popular diet plans, ask if we can be metabolically healthy without being skinny, and also examine the latest experimental data extolling the benefits of certain traditional diets, such as, for example, the Mediterranean diet. Finally, I will ask if recent genetic breakthroughs could really usher in an era of personalised diets perfectly tailored to our genes.

Understanding our genes and the biology of food intake is not simply an interesting academic exercise; it is essential, if we are to effectively tackle obesity and improve our health in the current food environment. Above all, particularly in the current 'post-truth' climate, it will be a defence, nay, a celebration of evidence-based science.

PART 1

A game of inches

You find out that life is just a game of inches.
So is football. Because in either game, life or football,
  the margin for error is so small . . .
The inches we need are everywhere around us.

Al Pacino, Any Given Sunday (1999)

CHAPTER 1

Are your genes to blame
when your jeans don't fit?

It has happened to us all.

You finally have a dinner date and you decide, in a fit of excitement, to call into service a pair of designer jeans you haven't worn in a little while. However, try as you may to pour yourself into the expensive denim, you find, to your horror, that the jeans now resemble a corset, requiring violent sucking in of your abdominal region, flirting with hypoxia, before the buttons can eventually meet the holes to perform their intended job.

Where can you ascribe blame for this scandalous state of affairs? Over-indulgence over the festive period? Your increasingly deskbound job? Above-inflation increases in your gym membership fees? Bankers? Or can you, as is seemingly fashionable, place the blame squarely at the feet of genetics? Are your genes to blame when your jeans don't fit?

To answer this question, it is worthwhile considering some numbers:

a) an average-sized woman should consume around 2,000 calories a day in order to survive, and an average-sized man 2,500 calories; or around 750,000 – 900,000 calories a year;

b) while ageing from a youthful, exuberant twenty years to a middle-aged fifty, an average person will, depressingly, typically gain 15kg (33lbs) in weight (some will of course gain little to no weight at all, while others will gain an awful lot more than 15kg);

c) if you or I were like a giant chocolate bar complete with nutritional information stamped on our collar labels, our caloric content would be around 5,000 calories per kg (give or take love handles/muffin-tops).

Because of c), the 15kg of weight gained over thirty years is worth about 75,000 calories, or 2,500 extra calories a year: a day's ration of calories if you're a man. If you did the necessary maths, you would find that an extra 7 calories a day for thirty years is all you would need to gain 15kg in weight!

Are you kidding me?

Other than it sounding like not an awful lot, what do 7 calories look like? Well, I rooted around my kitchen to see what I could find, and I came to the conclusion that nothing any of us would construe of as 'food' comes close to 7 calories. The nearest thing I could find was a 'serving' of ketchup. According to the nutritional information at the back of a half-empty squeezy bottle of ketchup that was purchased from a UK-based supermarket and languishing in my cupboard, a 'serving' of ketchup is 15g. Of course, to anyone who has ever introduced a bottle of ketchup to a burger or fries in anger, a 15g 'serving' of ketchup seems suspiciously austere. Even such a small amount of ketchup, however, would set back the energy storage account at the bank of your waistline a whole 15 calories. Using the same calculations as above, then the equivalent of an extra squeeze of ketchup, or even a heavy 'dip' with a chip or fry, every day for thirty years, would mean a weight gain of 30kgs!

The 'glass half empty' question that emerges from these numbers is: 'Why are we all not the size of houses?!' Good lord! We might all have to stop eating immediately, because of the imminent danger of exploding in a big red mess at the dining table! To the best of my knowledge, however, this is probably not happening out of sight in households up and down the country; at least certainly not on a regular basis.

Yet, when we reach for that extra chip, or helping of mayonnaise, or ketchup, or gravy, or wafer-thin mint, or a zillion other things which might be pleasant accompaniments to our meals but we don't even consider as real food, I guarantee that its energy content will be nearer to 70 calories than 7. So the 'glass half full' question is actually still, 'Why are we all not the size of houses?'

THE SET POINT

What is clear from data stretching back many decades is that mammals will robustly defend their bodyweight. The first data of this came not from humans, but from lab rats. Experiments done in the 1940s, which I have illustrated in the graph below, found that if a rat was left in a cage to its own devices and with sufficient food, it would grow at a certain rate. (Rodents, incidentally, never stop growing; they will keep growing until the day they die.) If the amount of food provided to the rat was reduced (i.e. if the rat was placed on a 'diet'), the rat would lose weight, which was unsurprising. Once the amount of food that was provided went back to normal however, the rats rapidly began to gain back the weight, but interestingly, only back to the growth rate they were on before the 'diet', and then they carried on like the diet never happened. When the food provided to the rats was changed to something very palatable, say high in sugar and fat, then the opposite was true, with their weight rapidly increasing. Once their food source was back to normal, the rats' weight drifted back down to the previous trajectory. These experiments led to the so-called 'set point' hypothesis, which proposed that all mammals in a stable environment will achieve a genetically determined trajectory of growth. Any deviation from this trajectory, as with the dieting rats above, will be defended.

Data collected since those initial experiments shows that the same phenomenon occurs in humans. Despite all the holiday periods, the resulting diets, illnesses, pregnancies and life's many other little surprises, only very unusually will anyone deviate more than 20 per cent in their adult bodyweight over a lifetime. This is why when you see someone often, on a daily or weekly basis for instance, you can rarely tell if they have lost or gained any weight. Yet we do tend to gain weight as we age. Why?

There are two major reasons. First, as we clear our twenties and go through our thirties and beyond, we begin to accumulate inefficiencies in our various organ systems, such that our metabolism begins to slow down. Sadly, while this slow-down occurs at different rates in different people, it will happen in all of us. Second, on average, we move less as we get older; for example, perhaps with seniority in our jobs, we end up with more paperwork, and we have less time to get to the gym. Yet we don't tend to eat that much less (if at all) as we age. So when you head back for your

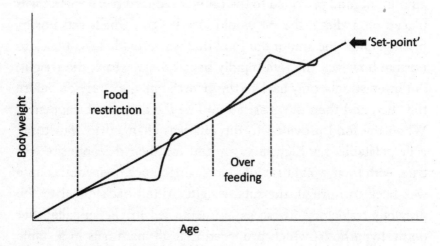

FIGURE 1 The 'set-point'

25th school reunion, you suddenly find it difficult to control your facial expression as you barely recognise anyone through all the increased fleshiness (I'm not trying to be a pot calling any kettle black as I would be unrecognisable as well).

The strategy used by our brain to defend our bodyweight is straightforward, even while the underlying mechanisms are complex (this will be a constant theme that runs through this book); that is, to influence food intake and energy expenditure. What I am not talking about here is the executive decision to go on a diet or to go to the gym. Those are conscious choices with their own distinct mechanistic and sociological underpinnings. Rather, the bodyweight defence strategy deployed by our brain is subconscious.

Let me give you an example. Imagine a typical festive season or some other vacation period, where there may have been a certain amount of overindulgence. Bacon and eggs every morning for breakfast you say? Sure! Desserts during both lunch and dinner? Why not! Eventually, and reluctantly, you have to get back to the real world and your normal day-to-day routine. Then comes that time in the day when you have to interact with food. Peering at a refrigerated supermarket shelf or perusing a menu in a restaurant, you may say, 'gosh, I don't feel so hungry tonight, I might just have a salad', thus eliciting a state of shock from your dinner companion.

I don't feel so hungry tonight.

Why not? Did you have a sudden attack of 'will-power'? Did a rod of steel just get shoved up your vertebral column, stiffening your back? No, the signals in your brain are simply making you feel 'not hungry'. 'Why can't I feel like that a little more often?' many of you will undoubtedly be thinking.

More than almost anything however, your brain absolutely hates it when you lose any weight. How much fat you are carrying is essentially how long you would last without food, so your brain equates weight loss to a reduced chance of survival. So when you lose even a few pounds, your body begins to fight back, making it rapidly more and more difficult (or so it seems) to shift each additional gram. Your body reduces its energy expenditure; it is with little consequence, for instance, that the energy efficiency of your metabolically most active organs, such as your liver or skeletal muscles, can be reduced by a few per cent. Your body also makes you feel more hungry, driving you to eat more. Keeping in mind that just a pesky 7 extra calories a day makes such a surprisingly large impact over a lifetime, the depressing phenomenon familiar to dieters the world over occurs; where after a couple of months, all of the weight you fought to lose has somehow grimly clawed its way back. This is, of course, what most will be familiar with as 'yo-yo' dieting, where you lose weight (yay!) then you regain the weight (boo!) and the cycle, depressingly, repeats itself interminably. Although it might seem as if you are gaining more weight than you had lost, this is seldom the case, and your weight will typically go back to where it was before you began your diet, i.e. your set point. Considering at any given point in time, nearly 20 per cent of you reading this book will be on some sort of 'diet', there are a lot of depressed people about due to this pattern.

BODY MASS INDEX

In fact, while 20 per cent of us are desperately trying to diet, the reality is that nearly 60 per cent of us in the UK and US are either overweight or obese.[1] Obesity is measured by Body Mass Index (BMI). This is a ratio of bodyweight in kilograms divided by the square of one's height in metres, and hence is represented as kg/m^2. A 'normal' BMI is $20-25kg/m^2$. Anything below a BMI of 18 would be considered underweight, a BMI of $25-30kg/m^2$ is considered 'overweight', and if you have a BMI north of $30kg/m^2$, you would then be classed as obese. However, it is important to know that ubiquitous as it is, BMI as a measure of 'fatness' is inherently imperfect because it is derived using purely your weight and your height. It cannot, for instance, differentiate between a rugby or American football player and a Joe Public of similar height and weight but carrying substantially less muscle mass. Crucially, it is the percentage of fat that one carries and where it sits in the body, rather than one's weight *per se*, that is strongly linked to disease.

There are any number of ways to measure fat percentage. The 'gold-standard' method of measuring fat-mass is by use of a technique called Dual-energy X-ray absorptiometry or DEXA. This is where two low-power X-ray beams, with different energy levels, are used to scan your body. X-Rays work by differentiating tissue density, which is why it is traditionally used to look at your bones, which are the densest part of the body. At a lower power however, it is also able to detect the difference between muscle (which has a higher density) and fat (which has a lower density), and therefore be used to calculate fat-percentage.

Another approach, that will be more familiar to many of you, will be the use of body-fat scales. These are available in countless models, and use a technology called 'bioelectrical impedance' to estimate how much body fat you have. The most popular models are integrated into traditional bathroom scales. When you step, barefoot, on to sensors on the scale, an imperceptible electrical current passes up one leg, across the pelvis and then down the other leg. There are also larger versions of these, typically built into weighing machines found in drug-stores or pharmacies, which get you to grip two handle-bars, and a current is passed through one arm, across your torso and through the other arm. The underlying principal in both these types of scales is identical. Because it contains much more water, muscle conducts electricity better than fat does, so the greater the electrical resistance, the more body fat you have.

But yet, in spite these available tools, the use of the BMI still dominates. Why is that?

DEXA is certainly both very accurate and precise. It is however, also expensive, requiring specialist equipment and technicians to run, so is just not logistically suitable for use in population-wide studies. The body-fat scales, while widely available, are notoriously inaccurate. There are too many variables, including how hydrated you are, when you last ate and exercised, and even whether your feet are particularly calloused or dirty, that can influence the calculated fat percentage from measurement to measurement. There is also the type and quality of the product itself, ranging in price from less than £30 to nearly £2,000, which precludes truly comparative measurements across different instruments.

In contrast, your BMI is free to calculate, assuming you have a way of weighing yourself and measuring your height, so is suitable for large population studies. And critically, despite being imperfect for measuring fatness in particularly athletic individuals, the sad fact is that the VAST majority of the population do not fall into this category. As a result, for most of us, the higher our BMI, the more fat we do tend to carry. So the use of the BMI as a proxy for 'fatness' continues to dominate.

IN AND OUT, IT'S PHYSICS!

Today, 60 per cent of us are carrying too much fat, making obesity one of the greatest public health challenges of the 21st century. It is a modern problem, with the prevalence of obesity having tripled in many countries in the world since the 1980s. According to the latest health report from the Organisation for Economic Co-operation and Development,[2] more than 30 per cent of adults in the US, New Zealand and Mexico, and more that 25 per cent in the UK, Australia, Canada, Chile, and South Africa, are obese. Within the European Union nearly 150 million adults and 15 million children are considered obese. The problem is not with obesity itself, but with the accompanying increased risk to a whole host of nasty diseases, including type 2 diabetes, heart-disease, high blood pressure and certain types of cancer. Unfortunately, we don't really have to gain that much weight before we are in the same frame as these 'co-morbidities'.

So how can we explain this rapid worldwide increase of bodyweight? Have our genes changed? Have we suddenly evolved? Clearly not. These dramatic changes have occurred over the past thirty years, against a constant gene pool and well within the lifetime of many of you reading this book. This would put the smoking gun in the guilty hands of 'environmental changes', an all-encompassing term used to describe changes in lifestyle, diet and working practices. Sadly, no matter how much one doth protest, the ONLY way you can gain weight, is if you eat MORE than you burn. It is simple physics.

Let me say this very clearly: the reason we have become more obese as a species is because we eat too much and don't move enough. Therefore, the only way to become less obese is to eat less and move more. There we have the cause and cure for the obesity epidemic. We all know this.

That being said, hidden in this simple statement is an oft-overlooked complexity that is well worth further exploration. Have a look at the two graphs below. Both indicate the real-world increase in average BMI, as charted by the US Centre for Disease Control or CDC, within the US population from 1985 ($23kg/m^2$) to 2014 ($27kg/m^2$).[3] The upper and lower graphs then plot two different possible distributions of BMI within the population in 2014 as compared to 1985. The upper panel models what the data would look like IF the environment was the ONLY influence on our bodyweight. In this scenario, everyone should respond to the environment in the same way, and everyone should therefore gain the same amount of weight. Thus the BMI distribution within the population should remain the same shape, but simply be shifted to the right, revealing a shape reminiscent of the Golden Gate Bridge.

The real data, however, shown in the bottom graph, reveals something very different. While the average BMI within the population has indeed increased, the shape of the 2014 curve has changed. This has happened because some people have gained lots of weight in the current environment, some not so much and some have not gained a single gram. In other words, everyone responds differently to the change in environment.

What all this means is that the environment cannot be the only thing that is influencing our BMI. There must be biological variation in our response to a changing environment. Put another way, the question of HOW we have become obese is one of physics. The question of WHY we have become obese requires examination of why some people eat more than others, why some people are more metabolically efficient and why some people burn more energy. It is in these latter questions that the biological variation lies.

Our biology, how we are put together, how our organs work, how the cells that characterise our organs function, how the molecules and proteins that form our cells interact, begins with our genes. So to understand biological variation, it is inescapable that we first need to understand variation in genetic heritability. The past twenty years of my life have been spent studying the genetic heritability of bodyweight and how it varies throughout the population.

THE POWER OF TWINS

One of the most invaluable tools in determining the genetic heritability of specific traits is the study of twins. Identical twins are genetic 'clones', while fraternal (or non-identical) twins share 50

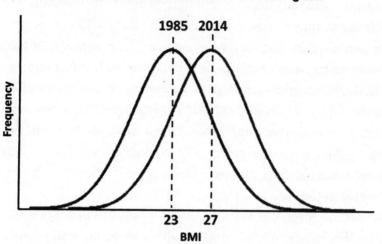

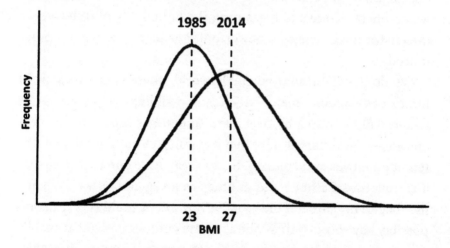

FIGURE 2 Two possible models to explain the increase in average BMI from 1985 to 2014

per cent of genetic material, as you would with any of your siblings. Thus, with the study of enough twins, both identical and non-identical, one could look at any trait that could conceivably have a genetic element, such as eye colour, hair colour, foot size, height or weight, and calculate how heritable each trait might be. As you might imagine, traits such as eye colour and hair colour (peroxide aside) are almost entirely genetically determined, with very little environmental influence. In contrast, while a trait like having freckles is clearly genetically influenced, whether, where and how many freckles appear will be down to how much time one spends in the sun.

There is, however, one valid argument against twin studies; that is, while the genetic power is self-evident, twins are still brought up in the same household, thus possessing a shared environment during their most formative of years. Surely this muddies the water when it comes to measuring the heritability of traits where the environment wields a powerful influence? A very good point indeed.

We do live in an unpredictable world where sometimes awful things can happen; one of which is that siblings, a percentage of whom will of course be twins, are sometimes separated at birth and raised in different adoptive homes, often in completely different countries and cultures. So you may have one twin raised as a carnivorous Catholic and another as a vegetarian Jew. When I first began my career, I did wonder how often could this situation possibly have occurred? While accurate numbers are not available, the answer is most certainly in the thousands – more often than any of us could ever imagine.

One, but by no means the only, driving force has been China's one-child policy, which has since been toned down somewhat. This led to the abandonment of tens of thousands of infants, amongst which were many hundreds of twin-pairs adopted and raised separately. Recently, there was a documentary by Norwegian filmmaker Mona Friis Bertheussen called *Twin Sisters*, telling the story of just such a pair of identical Chinese twin girls.[4] After being found abandoned in a cardboard box, Mia was adopted by a Californian couple and Alexandra by a couple from the north of Norway. Mia was raised as an 'all-American' girl, playing soccer, selling girl-scout cookies and going to the mall, while Alexandra led an outdoor life in the quiet solitude of a tiny village close to the Arctic circle. Just imagine the difference in diet and culture, in temperature and availability of sunlight, in education system and types of daily activity. Yet at ten years old when they eventually meet, aside from the expected language barrier, they are alike in character and temperament, and almost identical in height and weight. This same story has been reported many times over, with twins of other ethnicities and raised apart in other countries. Of course, the older the twins are when they are eventually reunited, the larger the influence of the environment, and consequently, the greater the variance in their weight. Time and time again, however, the power of genetics even in the face of such environmental differences is quite literally jaw-dropping.

What surprises most people is that the heritability of weight is actually close to that of height. No one would dispute the fact that height is genetically determined: tall parents = tall children. It is also well known that skeletons and written records show that human beings today are inches taller than humans just a century or two ago. For example, soldiers around the age of twenty who enlisted in the army during World War I were on average 168cm (5'6"), while today's average for young men is 178cm (5'10").[5] Why have we become taller as a species? Because of changes in diet, environment, and lifestyle.

It is the same argument with bodyweight, except that the changes have happened over a far shorter period of time. We are now more obese as a species compared to thirty years ago because of changes to our diet, environment and lifestyle. But it does not change the fact that if our parents are overweight and/or a certain shape, we are very much more likely to be overweight and/or be that shape. The studies demonstrated that the genetic heritability of bodyweight and shape in twins is approximately 70 per cent.[6]

The next time you have an opportunity to people watch, while you are at the airport or a coffee-shop for instance (please do be discreet), have a look at just how heritable body-shape in particular is. Your shape is largely determined by where fat sits in your body. This is not meant to depress you, but close your eyes for just one moment and reflect upon the shape of your parents. Does your mum have a big bum and a skinny upper body? Does your dad have a big tummy and skinny legs? Who do you look like? Who do your siblings look like? While the absolute amount of fat may differ – you may have a bigger bum or a smaller tummy, say – the chances are very high indeed that you will have the shape of one of your parents.

In truth, everything about us – our looks, our shape and size, our character, our intelligence, our athleticism, our risk of mental illness, even our risk of getting into a car accident, along with a million other traits – all have a genetic and an environmental component. It is very rarely, if at all, 100 per cent genetic or 100 per cent environmental. The real difficulty is in determining the relative contribution of each and, crucially, how they interact with each other.

DESERTS OF THE AMERICAN SOUTHWEST AND THE ISLANDS OF THE SOUTH PACIFIC

Yet another fact that has revealed the role of genetics in bodyweight is the observation that certain ethnic groups are more likely to become obese than others. Two examples from the more severe end of the spectrum have proven to be particularly informative.

The first are the Pima Indians, who are not South Asian Indians, but rather are indigenous or native Americans that live in the deserts of Arizona in the American Southwest. They are, infamously, one of the heaviest peoples in the world.[7] Nearly all Pimas, some from a frighteningly early age, become obese, with more than 50 per cent of Pimas suffering from type 2 diabetes.[8] This prevalence of type 2 diabetes is nearly five times higher than in the rest of the United States, a country of course deep in the grip of its own modern obesity crises. The Pimas, however, have been suffering from obesity and their related diseases for more than 50 years! And yet another group of Pimas, those living up in the Sierra Madre mountains of Mexico, display no proclivity to obesity at all. By all accounts, the Pima people were all initially from the Arizona region, but a contingent, at some point in the past and for some unknown reason, moved to the Sierra Madre. These two groups of Pima Indians remain genetically indistinguishable. Why, then, do they possess such vastly different bodyweights and rates of metabolic disease? The answer lies in the environment. The Arizona Pimas enjoy (is this the right word?) the American lifestyle, together with all of its conveniences and its excesses. The Sierra Madre Pimas however, still live like their ancestors. They are a farming community that still works with animals, with hard physical labour very much a part of everyday life, and who, of course, subsist on a very different diet from their American cousins. This is almost like having a time machine, allowing us to glimpse what the Arizona Pimas would have looked like living in the desert, prior to the arrival of European settlers.

The second example comes not from one singular ethnic group, but rather the multiple different peoples of the Pacific Island nations of Polynesia. The small island of Nauru for instance (and most of the Pacific Island nations are by and large small islands), is one of the most obese countries in the world, with nearly 95 per cent of its inhabitants being overweight and more than 45 per cent classed as obese. In fact, according to the World Health Organization (WHO), nine of the ten most obese countries or territories globally are Polynesian Pacific Islands.[9] The Cook Islands top this deadly leader board, with more than 50 per cent of their population classed as obese. Nauru, Palau, Samoa, Tonga and the Marshall Islands are all not far behind. This is, certainly when it comes to percentages, the fattest region in the world. Why is this the case?

On the face of it, the explanations that emerge when one takes a peek at Wikipedia or Google seem to make sense. One argument is that on these paradise islands, perhaps more than anywhere else in the world, there is wide cultural acceptance that bigger is more beautiful. Another argument, echoing the lifestyle issues faced by the Arizona Pimas, is that the life of the typical Polynesian is based upon consumption of imported, highly processed food, very little exercise and remote access to healthcare. These answers, however, are just too pat, too simplistic. Many cultures, for instance, embrace the 'big is beautiful' mantra, and a love of cheap processed food is hardly unique to the American Southwest and the South Pacific. But yet in an increasingly overfed world, these two groups of people stand out. What, then, are the root causes of these problems, and why have the results been so extreme for the Pimas and Polynesians in particular?

While the details differ, the underlying reasons are actually the same. In both regions, there have been millennia of adaptation to fluctuations of food availability in a harsh (for the Pimas) or geographically isolated (Pacific Islanders) environment and the necessity therefore of hard physical labour to secure food. Then quite abruptly, because of events completely out of their control, there was a very rapid and very dramatic change in the diet and lifestyle of both peoples.

The Pimas have lived on the banks of the Gila and Salt Rivers since long before European contact, which provided an important lifeline in the deserts of the Southwest. Life would have been very harsh, and a genetic premium would have been placed on those individuals better adapted to the episodic 'feast or famine' food environment. Those individuals who were better able to eat more and store fat during times of plenty and then be more efficient with energy usage in times of famine would have been more likely to survive. In turn, the genes which determined these survival characteristics were more likely to be passed on to their children. This is, in essence, evolution at play, with many generations of Pimas undergoing this extreme genetic selection, resulting in a population finely adapted to living in that particular environment. In the 1920s, however, the US government began a water irrigation project that necessitated the construction of a water storage dam on the Gila River upstream from Pima native lands, stopping its flow almost overnight. With the loss of their water (and thus food) supply, the Pimas became reliant on government food handouts. These tended to be processed, higher in sugar and refined flour and therefore much more calorically dense, and critically, a world away from their traditional diet. This mix of Pima genes with the new diet resulted in a rapid increase in levels of obesity.

Colonisation of the Polynesian Islands took place over nearly three millennia, beginning in the Philippines and New Guinea in around 1500 BC, Samoa in 800 BC, Hawaii and Easter Island not until 900 AD, with New Zealand the last to be colonised in 1200 AD. Given the geographic isolation of these tiny islands in an absolutely enormous area of the South Pacific, their colonisation is really a testament to human endeavour. The early Polynesians would first have had to survive canoe journeys of many weeks, and then, having arrived on small Pacific islands (atolls even), they would have to live and thrive. In this context, to be big meant certainly much more than being beautiful; it meant being much more likely to survive. The islanders formed – unsurprising given their geographic location – traditional fishing communities. The arrival of US and British airbases during World War II, as well as the proliferation of mining in some islands, drove globalisation, including the importation of western foods. These were brought in initially for the allied airmen and the miners. However, as is true the world over, imported food (highly processed in order to survive the journey) was very cheap and energy dense, and was rapidly embraced by the Polynesians. As with the example of the Pimas, the environment changed dramatically and rapidly for the Polynesians.

But why did both the Pimas and the Polynesians respond in such an extreme fashion to the change in environment? Many people, after all, you and me included, eat these same foods without tipping into extreme obesity. The difference is that the vast majority of us have adapted to live on continental plains. If our ancestors encountered a famine or drought, they could have mitigated against this 'selection pressure' and moved somewhere else. If, however, you were tied to one specific area like the Pimas, or were geographically isolated like the Polynesians, and therefore wouldn't or couldn't move, you either adapted quickly, or you died. Imagine, for a moment, if there was a sudden extreme change to our cosy situation that required us to be able to run really quickly, otherwise we would, say, be eaten by some rapidly reproducing carnivores with long legs and very pointy teeth. Well, we would very quickly end up with a population enriched with very fast run-ners, who would then pass on their genes to their offspring and so on and so forth. The fact that the Pima and Polynesian populations are still around meant that enough extraordinary individuals were able to adapt quickly, eating enough and storing enough fat during times of plenty, and being efficient during famines or paddling for weeks across the ocean, thereby surviving to pass those genes on. After just a few generations, those 'extraordinary' genes then became the norm within that population. The problem is that while those genes were advantageous and enabled survival in a 'feast–famine' environment, they have become deadly in today's 'feast–feast' environment.

All living creatures live by the golden rule to be as energy efficient as possible, in order to conserve calories for times of food austerity, and to make sure to eat as much as possible when the opportunity presents itself. So if a cheaper and more energy-dense food source suddenly appears, why would you continue wasting energy going out fishing or farming? That obviously had the deadly double result of increasing intake of highly calorific available foods (more about this later on in the book) and reducing physical activity in both the Pimas and Polynesians, thus driving the severe obesity problems in both communities.

THE HIGHLY EVOLVED RESPONSE

While the examples of the Pimas and Polynesians might seem extreme, the issues that arise are relevant to all of us. The concept of being as efficient with our energy expenditure and calorie usage as possible is true for us all. It is easy to forget that not so long ago, all our physical activity was gained from daily living. Working on the farms and in the mines; fishing and hunting; hand-washing everything (clothes and dishes); hand-sewing everything etc., etc. The whole concept of 'exercise' as a leisure activity would have been alien until just a few decades ago. Why would you do anything other than eat and sleep in your spare time, if you've spent all day in hard physical labour? If you think about it, is it not a weird thing for a significant chunk of the population to drive to a gym, maybe take an escalator or elevator up (or down) a couple of floors, only to get on a treadmill or stationary bike?

Then there is the current food environment we live in. One clear case in point is the phenomenon of 'fast food', which is, as we are all too familiar with, pervasive in our society. The vast majority of this food is calorically dense, highly processed, very cheap and often delivered straight to your door after a brief interaction with a smartphone.

What the data tells us is that, in effect, some of us simply feel a little more hungry all of the time. Not eating when you are not hungry is easy. Whatever the press, beauty/fashion/health/fitness magazines, Hollywood and 'inspirational I-did-so-you-can-too' speakers say, thin people are not morally superior, with the will-power of forged steel. They just feel a little less hungry, so get full up more easily. It requires no effort.

Have you, however, tried to stop eating when you are still hungry? It's difficult, even for one meal, because it's just not what we are designed to do. We have evolved to eat when we are hungry and when there is food, not to stop. Now imagine feeling slightly more hungry in this food environment and trying to halt the eating process every single day, for every single meal, for your whole life. This is what overweight and obese folk go through.

Obese people are not morally bereft, lazy or bad. They are fighting their biology. In fact, you could argue that being obese is the natural, highly evolved even, response to our 21st-century environment! We are simply preparing ourselves for a famine . . . that is never ever going to arrive.

But here is the rub. Not everyone has become obese in this environment. This is in contrast to our response to starvation, which is reassuringly uniform, across not only humankind but pretty much across the entire animal kingdom; that is, to find enough food as quickly as possible and eat it before you die. The dying bit ensured that only animals with the required drive and tools to find and eat food survived.

FROM GENETIC CODE TO FUNCTION

If you will indulge me, a brief genetics 'primer'. The complete set of our genetic material, our DNA, is called the genome. It is composed of three billion nucleotides, each coming in one of four different flavours; adenine or 'A', thymine or 'T', guanine or 'G' and cytosine or 'C'. Two complete sets of this genome (one from mum and one from dad) are present in every single cell in our body (the two exceptions being, depending if we are male or female, our sperm or eggs, which only contain one copy of the genome; and our red blood cells, which don't contain any DNA at all). DNA is literally a very long, thin thread of these three billion A, T, G and C nucleotides strung together. If it were possible to stretch out the DNA from a single cell, you would find it to be, incredibly, nearly two metres (six feet) long! This enormous length of DNA is tightly and neatly origamied into two sets of 23 different chromosomes (one set for each copy of the genome, so 46 chromosomes in total), each containing around 25,000 different genes. However, only 1–2 per cent of our three billion nucleotides in our genome actually code for genes. A significant but small percentage of the 98 per cent of 'non-coding' DNA are regulatory elements that control whether and how these genes are turned on or off. How much exactly we still don't know is the subject of ongoing and cutting-edge research. The vast majority of the remaining 'non-coding' DNA, what we used to call 'junk' DNA, remains 'dark' to us, and is largely a mystery. Much of this dark DNA may well turn out to be junk, but equally, there are almost certainly untold hidden treasures of functional significance yet to be uncovered.

The genes themselves do not confer function *per se*. Rather, they carry the information required to assemble the proteins that actually confer structure and function, the biology of life. Our genes are therefore an instruction manual for all of the different proteins that enable life.

ARE OUR GENES TO BLAME WHEN OUR JEANS DON'T FIT?

Mutations within our DNA happen randomly and at a low background level all of the time. Because the vast majority of our DNA has no known function, mostly these changes have no measurable effect. Rarely, a mutation may occur in a segment of DNA that regulates gene expression; meaning whether it is 'turned on', transcribed into RNA and translated into protein. Even more rarely, it could change the actual gene sequence, thus altering the function of the resulting protein. If the change in gene expression or sequence is severe enough to either disrupt translation or dramatically alter the function of its corresponding protein, it manifests as a disease, or at its most severe, death. At other times, however, genetic changes might simply modulate the function of the protein, either positively or negatively, depending on the environment.

If a genetic change is not desirable in a certain environment, then it is 'selected against' and not passed on. If a genetic change increases your chances of survival, then it is 'selected for' and that change is then passed on and integrates itself into the population. Take the response to starvation, for example. Any genetic change that increased your likelihood of finding enough food would mean that you could get bigger or faster or stronger, which would in turn increase your chances of finding a mate to reproduce and passing those genetic changes to your offspring.

Then there are genetic changes that in one environment have a neutral effect, but in another environment suddenly have a huge positive or negative effect. So, for example, in our current cosy situation, someone like Usain Bolt clearly runs very quickly and therefore can have a career in athletics, whereas while I cannot run quickly, I can make my living as a geneticist. Our proclivity to run has a neutral effect on our ability to survive in our current environment. But when the environment changes and long-legged pointy-toothed bitey carnivores begin to rapidly reproduce, Mr Bolt's fast twitch muscle genes suddenly have a positive effect on his ability to survive and are therefore selected for. In contrast, my ability as a geneticist has a neutral effect in the new environment, while my inability to run quickly has a negative effect on my likelihood of outrunning the carnivore.

Having too much food, coupled with not moving enough, is a contemporary problem, and would not have been a 'selection pressure' during evolution. With the rapid changes over the past few decades, accumulated genetic changes, which would have varied across the population and had a neutral effect when there was not enough food, were suddenly unmasked in our modern food and living environment. So while the average weight of the population has increased because everyone is exposed to more food and moving around less, some people, because of their repertoire of genetic variation, have become more obese than others in this environment.

So, to bring it back to my original question: are your genes to blame when your jeans don't fit? In many ways, yes. While the changing environment has undoubtedly driven the rapid increase in the prevalence of obesity, it is now becoming clear that our genes have influenced our response to this change. Where there are genes, there are molecules to identify and biology to study. That is what I am interested in studying; the pathways and mechanisms that control food intake, and how these vary between lean and obese individuals.

CHAPTER 2

It's all in your head

The Jackson Laboratory is a large facility where nearly 2,000 scientists work. It's an independent, non-profit biomedical research institution and has been a world centre for mouse genetics since 1929. One day in 1949, in a typical mouse cage, on one of the many racks, in one of the many rooms, a technician spotted an obese mouse. Not just a little tubby, perhaps needing to spend a little bit more time on the running wheel type of obese, but spherical; a mouse-coloured tennis ball with whiskers on one end, a tail on the other, and four paws.

A paper characterising these mice, which I dutifully dug out from the recesses of the internet, was published in the *Journal of Heredity* in 1950 by Ann Ingalls, Margaret Dickie and G. D. Snell from the Jackson Labs.[1] Using the colourful language of its time, under the section 'Description of Character' (case in point, the term 'character' in context of a mouse would just not be used today), the authors describe the mice as having 'a slightly shorter body, are rather square and have expansive hind quarters'. They proceeded to give this mouse the name 'Obese', which, I think you must agree, is a disappointing failure of imagination from the same minds that came up with 'expansive hind quarters'.

A second Jackson mouse of similar proportions, this time named 'Diabetes' was described by Katherine Hummel, Margaret (the one and very same) Dickie and Douglas Coleman in 1966.[2] Diabetes is a condition where you (and the vast majority of other mammals) lose control of blood glucose levels, which are normally tightly regulated by the hormone insulin. There are two major forms of diabetes: type 1, where damage to the pancreas means it stops producing insulin; and type 2, where the body slowly becomes resistant to the effects of insulin. Obesity is a major risk factor for type 2 diabetes. As it turns out, the 'Obese' and 'Diabetes' mice, both diabetic and reminiscent of mouse-coloured tennis balls, were actually identical in almost every way. In particular, they both ate voraciously (explaining their spherical geometry) and were both infertile, and it was apparent by the way these characteristics were inherited that these were the result of mutations in single genes.

GENETICS '101'

Most of us, when we were introduced to the concept of genetics at school, would have learnt about Mendel and his peas. Gregor Mendel, a 19th-century Augustinian friar and a scientist, is widely considered to be the father of modern genetics. He worked out the basic principles of genetics by breeding pea plants and observing how seven different characteristics (plant height, pod shape and colour, seed shape and colour, and flower position and colour) were inherited. Each of these characteristics happened to be determined by single genes. So let's take seed colour, for instance, which came in two flavours, yellow or green. When Mendel crossed 'true-bred' yellow-coloured pea plants (the pea colour was always yellow) with 'true-bred' green-coloured pea plants (see Cross 1 in figure 3 on the next page), he always got plants with yellow-coloured peas. There were no green-coloured peas at all. The key part of the experiment, and how he figured out what was happening, came

Mendelian Genetics

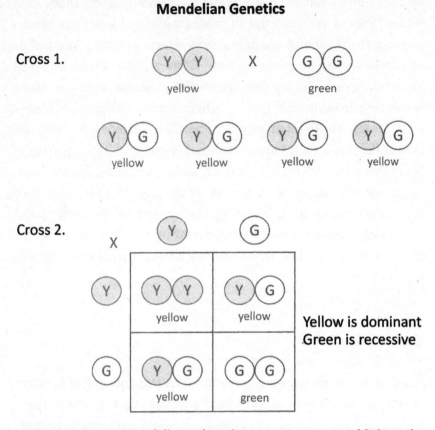

FIGURE 3 Gregor Mendel's pea-breeding experiments, establishing the concept of dominant and recessive genes

when he bred the yellow offspring from the first cross together (Cross 2 in the figure). What he found was that three-quarters of the offspring from this second cross were yellow, while the green-coloured peas re-appeared, but only in one quarter of the offspring. He saw similar results in all of the seven characteristics that he was studying.

He deduced two fundamental principles from these breeding experiments. First, he worked out that each of the pea plant's traits had to be determined by two copies of some invisible factor: these would later be called 'genes', one coming from each parent plant. Second, some of these genes would be 'dominant' and others 'recessive'. Yellow was dominant over green because a single copy of the yellow gene meant yellow-coloured peas. Whereas a pea would only be green if it carried two copies of the green gene, thus green was 'recessive'. While it is true that most traits are not determined by single genes but by a combination of genes, these basic principles still govern how we consider genetics and heritability today.

'OBESE' AND 'DIABETES': DIFFERENT MUTATIONS IN DIFFERENT GENES

So with the above information in mind, let's revisit our mice in the Jackson lab. The scientists knew that 'Obese' and 'Diabetes' were the result of single genes because the obesity in both these lines of mice was always linked to the infertility, while the parents were never obese and (by definition) fertile. What this had to mean was the parents each carried one copy of the mutation (or to be heterozygous, like in Cross 2 of Mendel's pea experiment) and only when offspring inherited two copies of the mutation (to be homozygous, like the green peas), one from each parent, do they become obese and infertile. This is therefore a 'recessive' type of inheritance.

So if both 'Obese' and 'Diabetes' were identical in nearly every way, did they perhaps carry a mutation in the same gene? Keep in mind that this was before the era of modern genetic techniques, so aside from working out that it was likely to be a single mutated gene in each case and that it was recessively inherited, nothing else was known. To answer this question, Doug Coleman went about performing what can only be described as odd 'parabiosis' experiments to try and work this out. Parabiosis is where you stitch two

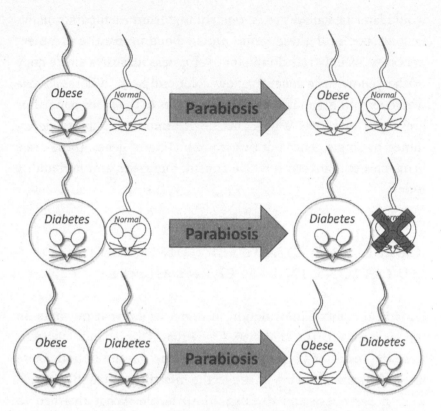

FIGURE 4 Doug Coleman's 'parabiosis' experiments that led to his 'satiety' factor hypothesis

mice together, so they end up sharing their blood circulation, sort of a reverse Siamese twin surgery. It was not for the faint of heart and is, to be clear, no longer done today. But these were different times.

Doug performed three parabiosis experiments. First, he stitched an obese mouse to a normal mouse-sized mouse. What he saw was that while nothing happened to the normal-sized mouse, the obese mouse lost a great deal of weight. In the second experiment, he attached a diabetes mouse to a normal-sized mouse. This time, intriguingly, the normal-sized mouse stopped eating, lost weight and eventually wasted away, whereas nothing happened to the diabetes mouse, who continued eating and did not lose any weight. In the third experiment, Doug paired the obese and diabetes mice together. What happened was like in the first experiment; the obese mouse stopped eating and began to dramatically lose weight, whereas, like in the second experiment, there was no change to the diabetes mouse.[3] Hmmmm ... curiouser and curiouser.

Well, the most obvious thing that these experiments told us was that the Obese and Diabetes mice had mutations in different genes, because they each behaved differently when stitched to the average-sized mice and to each other. Less obviously (certainly to me, at least), was the conclusion that Doug drew. Doug proposed that the Obese mouse was lacking a 'satiety' factor that would normally be circulating in the bloodstream, stopping the mouse from eating when its levels were high, whereas while the diabetes mouse had the circulating 'satiety' factor, it was unable to respond to it. I know ... it does seem an extraordinary conclusion to draw from the results. But I'll take you through Doug's logic. In the first experiment, when the Obese mouse was attached to the average-sized mouse, it was suddenly exposed to the circulating satiety factor in that mouse. As a result, the Obese mouse stopped eating and began to shrink. In the second experiment, because the diabetes mouse was resistant to the notional satiety factor, its body responded by producing sky-high levels of the factor to counteract the resistance, so that when the unsuspecting average-sized mouse was attached, it responded to the enormously raised signal by immediately ceasing to eat, leading to its untimely demise. The final experiment, where the Obese and Diabetes mice were attached to each other, convinced Doug that the mutated genes in the two mice interacted with each other, because the high circulating levels of the satiety factor in the diabetes mouse flowed into the obese mouse, which lacked it, thereby causing it to stop eating.

That at least, was the hypothesis. Now there was only the small matter of it needing to be tested.

LEPTIN: THE 'HUNGRY GENE'?

It wasn't, however, until the mid-1980s, with the advent of rapidly developing genetics techniques, that a team from the Rockefeller University in New York initiated a programme of research that made real progress in testing this hypothesis. Finally in 1994, forty-five years after it was first noticed sitting in a cage, the lab of Jeffrey Friedman reported that the obese mouse had a mutation in a gene that Jeff coined *leptin*.[4]

Leptin, as it turns out, is made in fat and is secreted into the bloodstream, where it circulates like a hormone. When Jeff made leptin and injected it back into an obese mouse, it stopped eating and shrank dramatically, confirming that it was indeed the lack of functioning leptin that gave the obese mouse its eponymous rotund characteristic. This was the long missing 'satiety factor' of Doug's prediction. A couple of years later, the diabetes mouse was found to have a mutation in the receptor for leptin and, unlike its obese counterpart, did not shrink when given leptin.[5] So once again, Doug's prediction – that the diabetes mouse had the 'satiety factor' (leptin), which was missing from the obese mouse, flowing through its bloodstream but was unable to respond to it – was, remarkably, entirely accurate!

The identification of leptin and its receptor showed, for the first time, that there was a hormone system that could regulate food intake, and that it wasn't simply an issue of willpower. But then came the next important question. Was this some weird system found only in mice, or did it have broader applicability in other mammals as well? It was at this point, early in 1997, that my long-time colleagues Stephen O'Rahilly and his (at the time) clinical fellow Sadaf Farooqi entered the story. Remember that the obese mutation in the leptin gene was not genetically engineered, but a naturally occurring phenomenon. Steve, a moustachioed Irishman partial to musing, mused that if a mutation in a gene could cause obesity in one mammalian species, surely it could also happen in humans? In one of the freezers in his department, Steve had blood samples from two kids who were first cousins and were both severely obese. Sadaf tried to measure leptin in these samples and failed. To be more accurate, she didn't fail; rather, the assay didn't detect any leptin in either sample. Then Carl Montague, who was Steve's post-doctoral fellow, sequenced the leptin gene in these children, and found a mutation, a deletion of a single guanine or 'G' (guanine is one of the four alphabets that make up the DNA code; the other three being adenine or 'A', thymine or 'T' and cytosine or 'C') in both cousins. The consequence of the deletion of this single 'G' meant the absence of a functioning leptin protein. Steve's musing was (not for the first time or the last) correct. His team at the University of Cambridge had just found, for the first time, that a mutation in a single gene could result in severe obesity in humans.[6]

So what did these kids who could not produce leptin look like? Well, the younger of the two cousins was a boy of three years old, let's call him John B, who weighed 42kg (92.4 lbs). For some perspective, I weigh 75kg (165 lbs). So here was a three-year-old who was two-thirds my weight. This is not 'PlayStation' obesity; not a case of drinking one too many cans of fizzy soft-drinks; something was clearly very wrong with this child. John B was born at a normal birthweight; however, when he moved from milk to solid food, something dramatic began to occur. He became very, very hungry. He was 'hyperphagic', with no preference for any particular food. From Latin, *hyper* means 'more' and *phagic* means 'eat', so 'more eat'. This describes an abnormal eating behaviour. For instance, you can't say, 'boy, I was hyperphagic last festive season' or, 'gosh, a severe bout of hyperphagia struck me during that weekend trip to Greece' – you just ate too much. Hyperphagia means that these kids had to have their freezer doors padlocked, because otherwise they would get in and eat frozen fish fingers. I can already hear your reaction: ewwwwww! Perhaps unsurprisingly, both kids had a really high body-fat percentage of around 57 per cent, where normally one would expect, depending on whether you are male or female, a level of 15–28 per cent. What was unexpected was that the older cousin, let us call her Jane A, had not gone through puberty (John B was, at the time, too young for puberty to have been an issue) and both had impaired immune systems. At first glance, theirs seems an odd combination of characteristics . . . obese, weird eating behaviour, infertile and a wobbly immune system. However, I am going to come back to this later and show you how this isn't actually weird at all, but ends up making perfect sense . . . yes, even the eating of frozen fish fingers.

People with type 1 diabetes do not produce any of the hormone insulin and as a result have to inject themselves multiple times a day with insulin in order to control their blood-sugar levels. So, these children who don't have leptin circulating in their blood, can they replace it in a similar way? This was the next question that Steve and Sadaf tackled. When the children were injected with leptin, they, in almost miraculous fashion, suddenly didn't feel hungry any more and began to lose weight. After daily injections of leptin, John B, who as I said was 42kgs at three years old, continued to grow taller and yet shrank in width at the same time, such that by the time he turned into a seven-year-old boy, he weighed a perfectly normal 32kgs. Greater than 95 per cent of the weight that was lost was fat. The leptin patent was owned by Jeff Friedman's home institution, the Rockefeller University, but was licensed at the time to the American pharmaceutical giant Amgen. Oh to have been a fly on the wall at one of their boardroom meetings when those results came out. They must have been wetting themselves, thinking that all of their Christmases had arrived in one big 'show me the money' moment. We have cured obesity! Woohoo!

Except of course, they hadn't. The paper in the New England Journal of Medicine by Sadaf, Steve and colleagues describing these findings was published in 1999.[7] Leptin was given to many different people: men, women and children of all different ages, ethnicities and sizes.[8] The bottom line was this: it didn't matter what BMI you were, whether you were the size of a supermodel like Kate Moss or if you were the size of Santa Claus. As long as you had a functioning leptin system, then you did not respond to any extra leptin, at least in terms of food intake. Why would this be the case, given the dramatic results when leptin was given to someone who did not have leptin? As I mention above, leptin is made in fat and released into the bloodstream, so the more fat you carry, the more leptin you will have. Perhaps because of its genesis, emerging as it did from Doug Coleman's concept of a missing 'satiety factor' in the obese mice, 'leptin' actually came from the Greek word *'leptos'*, meaning thin. At the time, most people in the field, myself included, just thought that leptin functioned in a classical 'negative feedback loop', meaning if you ate too much you would get fat, which would raise leptin levels, and leptin would then signal to your brain to get you to eat less; this would in turn lower fat levels and therefore leptin, making you eat more again, and so on and so forth. The fact that when you gave leptin to the kids with no leptin and they ended up feeling less hungry and losing lots of weight appeared to support this hypothesis. However, if you look at this with a bit more of a critical eye, you begin to see that it does not make a great deal of sense. Leaving aside the last thirty years or so, when else in human history would we have had enough to eat, such that too much fat would become a problem? Never is the answer. The truth is, we never had enough food, so there would have been no selection pressure on us and our genes to develop a system to stop us from eating too much.

LEPTIN: THE STARVATION HORMONE

As it turns out, and so very elegantly demonstrated by Jeff Flier's group at Harvard, leptin does not function when there is too much of it, but rather when there is not enough of it.[9] One of leptin's most important roles is to inform your brain how much fat you have. This is an important piece of information and not only because it impacts on whether or not you can fit in your jeans. Fat, after all, is your long-term energy store, so crucially, how much fat you are carrying is directly related to how long you would last without food. Not having enough leptin means not having enough fat, and not having enough fat means you are starving. Leptin is not, as Doug Coleman hypothesised, a satiety signal; rather, it is a starvation hormone. During a prolonged period of time without sufficient food, and as your fat stores begin to dwindle, leptin levels in the blood plummet, which turns on the 'starvation response'.

What is the starvation response? Well, the first thing is clearly to find food to eat. We all know that when we are really hungry, even a slice of bread or a bit of rice or pasta tastes like heaven. However, as we get less hungry, we get far fussier about our food. Imagine if you were ACTUALLY starving, though; plane-crash-in-the-Andes, your-partner-is-beginning-to-look-delicious type of starving; would YOU eat frozen fish fingers to keep yourself alive? Of course you would.

Your brain, which is the 'command and control' centre, is possibly the most energy-expensive organ in our body. It weighs just 2–3 per cent of our total bodyweight, yet, at rest, it uses up 25 per cent of the glucose in our blood. So the second thing that happens is your body begins to triage nutrients to preserve fuel for your brain, in order to ensure that even in your haze of hunger, you are actually able to pull together a coherent strategy to find food. It does this by shutting down immediately unnecessary and metabolically expensive functions. One of these is reproduction. Ladies in particular, you know that every month during menstruation there are a lot of wasted calories, which when you are close to the edge of starvation, or actually starving, can be the difference between life and death. Also, if you are starving, the last thing you would want to do is to plop a baby out onto the Serengeti, as an environment lacking in food is clearly one not ideal in which to try and keep a squawking bundle of joy alive. As a consequence, your body simply turns reproduction off. Another metabolically expensive function that is 'tuned down' is the immune system. Your immune system can be imagined as a whole collection of 'pilot lights', one for each bug or virus encountered through your life, ready to flare up at a moment's notice like the 'bat signal' over Gotham City, calling into action your body's defences should any one reappear. 'But won't I die of an infection?' I hear you ask. Well, since this is a triage situation and the immediate danger is dying of starvation, your body prioritises your brain over your immune system.

So whilst clearly displaying all of the visible hallmarks of being severely obese, because both Jane A and John B had no leptin, there was no way for their brains to sense the amount of fat stores available and they were as a consequence, for all intents and purposes, in starvation mode. Crucially, leptin does not only turn the starvation response 'on' as its levels drop, it also turns it back 'off' again when levels begin to rise. When the leptin-deficient patients are treated with leptin, the most immediate effect is the abeyance of hyperphagia, resulting eventually in dramatic weight loss, as demonstrated clearly above. In terms of reproduction, Jane A, nearly twenty years on from first being treated with leptin, has just had her first child; the first leptin-deficient person in human history to reproduce. And while I did not go into the details, the immune systems of both children were also normalised. Hyperphagia, infertility and a wonky immune system, all fixed once leptin was reintroduced.[10]

Lest you think that this phenomenon is unique to leptin being injected, consider women who, for one reason or another, have very little body-fat. They could be catwalk models or suffering from eating disorders such as anorexia, or they could even be elite female endurance athletes. The latter are spectacularly fit and the former are unhealthily skinny, but women from both groups very often menstruate irregularly or even not at all. For the athletes this condition is referred to as Athletic Amenorrhea. A key driver for this is the very low levels of body-fat and consequently the very low leptin levels, which are then shutting down reproductive function, for the reasons I have discussed above. The easiest way for these women to fix the problem is actually to gain weight!

Mutations in the leptin gene causing severe obesity are still vanishingly rare, with only 30–40 families identified worldwide as having the condition since 1997. However, the biological insights we have obtained from studying this rare condition have been enormous. It has opened our eyes to a whole new biological system that plays a central role in how our brain controls food intake, which is what much of the rest of this chapter is going to focus on.

GUT FEELING

Thanks in large part to the discovery of leptin, we now know that there are hormones that circulate in the blood and signal to the brain, letting it know the nutritional status of the body. Broadly speaking, there are two sources for these signals. The first is hormones secreted from fat, which are, as I have discussed above, our long-term energy stores. Of these, leptin is arguably the most important, but many others do exist, although I won't go through all of them here.[11]

However, in order to effectively modulate your feeding behaviour, your brain not only needs to know how long you would last without food, it also needs to know what you are currently eating and what you have just eaten. Thus, the second source is short-term signals secreted from our stomach and gut.

Every time we take a mouthful of food, from the moment we begin chewing, till the moment it emerges from the other end, hormones are secreted at every step of the way. Incidentally, I do a demonstration to primary school children, involving a marble and a full-sized knitted gut (with thanks to the mothers of the 'Anglesey in Stitches' knitting group), which I call our 'food to poop tube'. It is incredibly popular with the kids (and quite a few of the teachers), primarily because I say the word 'poop' multiple times . . . yup, it's all fun and games here in Cambridge! But I digress. As food makes its way through our gastrointestinal tract, hormones are released all along the way that reflect not only how many calories are in the meal, but also its 'macronutrient content', that is, how much protein, fat and carbohydrates are present. We might for instance, while sitting in a Korean BBQ joint, visibly recognise that the meal placed in front of us was soy-sauce-marinated sirloin steak grilled medium rare, served with steamed rice and (for all you lovers of spicy fermented cabbage) kimchi. However, any 'guesstimate' about the caloric or macronutrient content of the meal would be just that, a guess. In contrast, your secreted repertoire of gut hormones following the meal would reflect that you've had 300 calories of animal-based protein, 200 calories of fat, 500 calories of complex carbohydrates, and 200 calories of fibre and cellulose. One calorie of carbohydrate or one calorie of fat is easier to digest than one calorie of protein; cellulose we can't digest at all, and passes right through. In very broad terms, the more difficult and longer something takes to digest, the farther down the gut it will travel, resulting in different hormones being secreted. We are going to spend a lot more time on the gut, the different hormones that it releases and how it handles different foods later on in the book.

CENTRAL COMMAND AND CONTROL

Whether long-term signals secreted by fat or short-term hormones emerging from the stomach and gut, it is the brain that integrates these signals and influences our feeding behaviour at the next meal. There are two key parts of your brain that play a role in this integration; there is the brain-stem, which is where your brain meets your neck; and then, pretty much right in the centre of your head, at about the level of the bridge of the nose, is a part of the brain, about the size of your thumbnail, called the hypothalamus. The hypothalamus is important for many functions, including regulating body temperature, sleep cycles and thirst, amongst many others. Another key function, which is relevant to our discussion here, is its role as our 'fuel sensor'. Briefly (and do forgive me for all the acronyms for now, but all will soon be made clear), leptin, reflecting the amount of fat, circulates through the blood and signals to the leptin receptor on, amongst many others,

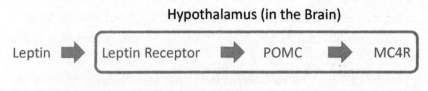

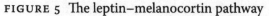

FIGURE 5   The leptin–melanocortin pathway

POMC neurons in the hypothalamus. This leads to the release of small fragments of POMC called melanocortin peptides, which go on to signal to another population of neurons that express the MC4R, thereby influencing food intake. This is the so-called 'leptin–melanocortin pathway', which is the best-characterised and, as far as we know, one of the most critical circuits in the brain that senses fat and controls appetite. In fact, genetic mutations at every stage of this pathway (in mammals and other vertebrates) result in increased food motivation and obesity. I (together with many others in the obesity field) have spent twenty years studying many different aspects of this circuit, and many books could be written exclusively on the subject.[12] Instead, in the interest of brevity and not boring most people silly, I will discuss just a few examples that highlight the importance of this pathway in modulating not only our (humans') feeding behaviour, but also those of many other creatures great and small.

PROOPIOMELANOCORTIN (POMC)

A veterinary-surgeon colleague of mine, Eleanor Raffan, did her PhD studies in human genetics in our institute, but then went back, understandably, to becoming a vet. Eleanor has always been interested in Labrador retrievers, which are the most popular pet-dog breed in the UK and North America. 150,000 new Labrador puppies are registered every year here in the UK alone! They make for a lovely family dog because of their temperament. However, as all Labrador owners know, don't leave compost bins or any other type of container with edible items in it open, otherwise the dog will try, and often succeed, in eating everything in said container. Not good for your compost, your edible items or indeed, your Labrador, who could literally eat till their stomach was close to popping. Labradors are well known to be very food motivated indeed and are therefore prone to obesity, which is of course what interested Eleanor and me about them.

Before deploying the latest genetic tools and tricks to unpick the Labrador obesity puzzle, we started by just looking at genetic variation around the melanocortin pathway. Now, many people don't admit this, but serendipity often plays a significant role in scientific breakthroughs, as it did here. Lo and behold, in just the second gene that she looked at, Eleanor found that about a quarter of Labradors have a deletion in the POMC gene![13]

Proopiomelanocortin is the full, unabridged name for POMC, the important takeaway being 'melanocortin', which gives its name to the eponymous pathway. It is made as one large complex 'pro-protein' that is then subsequently processed and chopped into a number of smaller fragments called the melanocortin peptides (see illustration below). These peptides signal to five different melanocortin receptors (MC1R–MC5R) to mediate quite a dizzying array of biological functions.[14] So, for example, while a person's ethnicity is clearly the primary determinant of skin and hair colour, the MC1R plays a powerful modulatory role, such that when melanocortin peptides bind to the MC1R, you get a darker pigmentation and when they don't, you get a lighter pigmentation. As a result, common variations (known as polymorphisms) in the MC1R gene are associated with normal differences in skin and hair colour, with certain MC1R polymorphisms found most commonly in folks with red hair, very fair skin, freckles, and an inability to go out in the sun without first applying factor 100 sunblock. The MC2R is required for the proper development of the adrenal gland, which is important in steroid production and response to stress. The MC3R and MC4R are both found in the brain, with the MC4R in particular playing a key role in control of appetite; it gets its own section below. The MC5R has an important function in maintaining the natural oils (known as sebum) secreted by the skin.

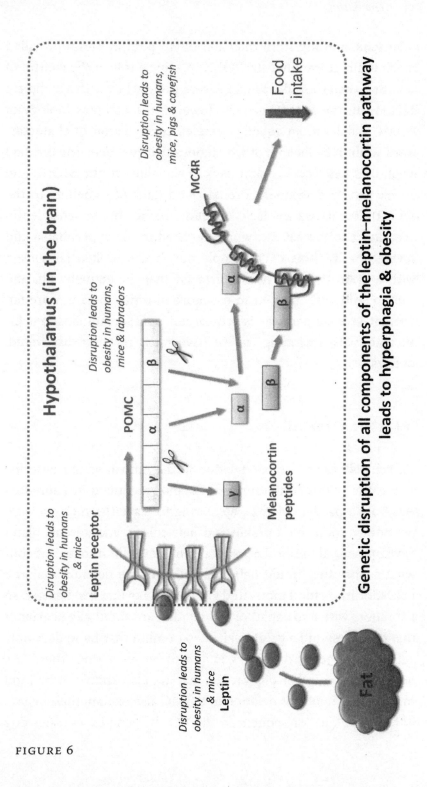

FIGURE 6

In 1998, a group from the Charité Hospital in Berlin provided the first direct evidence for POMC playing a role in the control of appetite when they identified a severely obese boy with a complete deletion in the POMC gene.[15] However, the complex biology of POMC results in an equally complex constellation of characteristics when it is deleted, of which obesity is just one. The boy had bright red hair and fair skin (lack of signalling to the MC1R) and a very poorly developed adrenal gland (lack of signalling to the MC2R). But it was the lack of POMC being able to sense leptin and signal to the MC4R, which resulted in his hyperphagia and severe obesity. This child, simply put, had a broken fat sensor, with a brain thinking he had less fat than he actually did, and consequently driving him to eat more in order to gain more fat. This fat-sensing pathway is critical not only for humans, but for all mammals, including, as we have most recently discovered, in dogs.

'FLABRADORS'

Unlike the near complete deletion in the human gene I describe above, the POMC mutation that Eleanor identified in Labradors was only a partial deletion, appearing to leave the melanocortin peptides responsible for skin and hair colour, and adrenal gland development alone, so Labradors don't have an orange coat (but what a sight that would be!). Each copy of the deletion makes a Labrador more food motivated and nearly 2kg (4.4 lbs) heavier; so Labradors with two copies of the deletion are about 4kg heavier. If that doesn't sound a great deal, keep in mind that Labradors only get to about 30–35kg, so 4kg is quite a bit more dog. There are, however, many other dog breeds that are also known to be food motivated. Might this deletion in POMC also explain their behaviour? Well, Eleanor sequenced the POMC gene in 38 other dog breeds, from Chihuahuas and Yorkshire Terriers, to Greyhounds and Great Danes; nearly all had a normal POMC. The only exception was the Flat-Coated Retriever, which is the breed most closely related to the Labrador Retriever. Flat-Coated Retrievers are a lot rarer than Labradors, with about 1,500 new puppies registered a year here in the UK, which is why many of us, myself included, would probably have trouble pointing one out. Flat-Coats have the exact same mutation in POMC, and like Labradors, it makes them more food-motivated and prone to obesity. So how did this mutation find its way into these two dog breeds? Labradors and Flat-Coats are both descended from the now extinct St John's Waterdog, which were bred between the 17th and 19th centuries in Canada, to accompany Newfoundland fishermen in their boats and retrieve lines or nets of fish, hauling them back to the boat. You might imagine that one day a few hundred years ago, a burly fisherman with a big beard, while selecting dogs for breeding to jump into the icy-cold waters off Newfoundland, might have noticed a particularly well-padded dog (more insulation) who was willing to work harder for food (as motivation). Unbeknownst to anyone at the time, that dog just happened to carry the deletion in POMC, making it a superior waterdog, and thus the mutation was selected for and kept within the population, eventually passing it on to Labradors and Flat-Coats.[16]

In addition to their lovely disposition and temperament, another reason Labradors are such popular dogs is their trainability. In fact, these defining characteristics explain why they are overwhelmingly used as guide dogs for the blind in the UK and North America. These dogs are like the 'navy seals' of the dog world, highly selected for and trained within an inch of their lives, because they are about to be given a blind person to look after for the rest of their working lives. The relevant thing here is that they are very often trained with food, using standard Pavlovian approaches. It was therefore intriguing when we studied one group of Labrador guide dogs, that in contrast to pet Labradors, nearly 80 per cent of them carried the genetic mutation! Imagine if a guide dog was leading visually impaired Mr Smith along, and suddenly a chicken runs across the road (it could happen!). Now what are the chances of successfully procuring a chicken dinner? Maybe 20 per cent at best? Whereas the guide dog has been trained to know that there is a 100 per cent chance he will get food if he manages to chaperone Mr Smith safely to his destination. We think that in the group of guide dogs we studied, those carrying the POMC deletion have been heavily selected for because of their genetically driven motivation towards food, which has, in effect, manifested into having a desirable temperament and being receptive to training (with food). The press, worldwide, loved this story, with coverage in all of the major print and broadcast outlets ... Who knew that fat Labradors would elicit such interest! One of the UK tabloid papers came up with my favourite tagline: 'Flabradors: Family favourite breed most likely dog to beg for food and overeat due to a "faulty fat gene", say boffins'. Much to like about this, from the ever so slightly non-PC moniker 'Flabradors' (but I guess we are talking about dogs), to being referred to as a 'boffin'.

So next time your Labrador looks at you with those big googly puppy-dog eyes, nuzzling you with his wet nose, and you think 'awwwww, Fido loves me!' . . . he doesn't love you, he is hungry!

MC4R

I had just completed my PhD in Genetics at the University of Cambridge early in 1998 and after years of bumming around as a student, I was finally looking for gainful employment. My PhD project had been on the molecular evolution of immune related genes in the Japanese pufferfish *Fugu Rubripes*, which was, to put it mildly, quite niche. To expand my job opportunities, I thought it wise to cast the net (pun intended) beyond just pufferfish. DNA, after all, is DNA, whatever life form it comes from, thus I was agnostic about the species I would be working on. I hawked myself, from lab to lab, as a well-trained molecular geneticist, which, if I'm to be perfectly honest, had far less to do with me than my PhD supervisor Sydney Brenner, who picked up the Nobel Prize in Physiology and Medicine in 2002. One of the lab doors I knocked on was that of Steve O'Rahilly. It was only a scant six months or so since the publication of the landmark paper characterising the first leptin-deficient patient, and Sadaf had begun the process of recruiting more severely obese kids, to see what other obesity genes might exist. So as luck would have it, Steve was in the market for a geneticist, and I was the right person, in the right place, at the right time, and before I knew it, I became a newly minted post-doctoral researcher at the University of Cambridge.

On literally my first day on the job, Steve mused to me (he is, as you might recall, partial to musing) that evidence was accumulating that implicated the melanocortin 4 receptor (MC4R) in regulating appetitive behaviour, and that I should start by screening the gene in the rapidly growing cohort of severely obese kids. So off I went, and a few months later found a mutation in the MC4R gene in a severely obese boy and his rather large father (Steve's musing was, once again, startlingly accurate), which resulted in my first significant publication.[17]

Aside from severe obesity, there are some important differences between someone with a deficiency in MC4R and a similarly sized person lacking leptin:

a) leptin deficiency is a recessive condition, whereas MC4R deficiency is dominant, with a mutation on one copy of MC4R sufficient to result in hyperphagia and obesity;

b) whereas leptin patients are of average height, MC4R-deficient patients are almost always very tall (the dad from my first publication, for example, was over 2m [6'7"]);

c) while the MC4R-deficient patients are the same weight as those with leptin deficiency, they don't carry as much fat (43 per cent fat as compared to 57 per cent in leptin deficiency), which means they have more muscle;

d) and finally, MC4R deficiency does not impact on the ability to reproduce.

As a consequence of (a) and (d), mutations in MC4R are far more commonly found than mutations in leptin, or the leptin receptor or indeed POMC. It turns out, at least to date, to be the commonest single gene cause of obesity, with 5–6 per cent of Sadaf's cohort of several thousand severely obese kids (of similar size to the leptin-deficient children) having 'loss of function' mutations in MC4R.[18] In fact, it is estimated that 1 per cent of people with a BMI greater than 30, have a mutation in MC4R.[19] Put another way, 1 per cent of people are obese because of MC4R deficiency; so in the USA, where nearly 100 million people are obese, that is around 1 million (tall) people with mutations in MC4R.

THE MELANOCORTIN PATHWAY INFLUENCES FOOD INTAKE AND PREFERENCE

Mutations in MC4R are not localised to one specific part of the receptor, but rather they span the entire gene. Unsurprisingly, some of the more severe mutations – deletion, for example – resulted in a receptor with no ability to respond to melanocortin peptides, while the more subtle mutations resulted in receptors with anywhere from 30–70 per cent loss of function. In order to study how the various mutations influence the amount of food eaten, Sadaf (now Professor) Farooqi devised a breakfast test buffet, which contained an incredible 4,300 calories. This test really only works on children, because imagine if an adult, and an obese adult at that, came into a room with that much food, and was asked to 'eat naturally' whilst being watched: they would be self-conscious and the experiment would not work. And the reason such a ridiculous amount of food is used is to make sure that it is impossible for the children to eat it all. Alongside studying the children carrying mutations in a variety of genes (MC4R in this situation), 'control children', or non-obese children, were also tested in the buffet. These tended to be, because of proximity and ease of recruitment, offspring of scientists and clinicians in the institute. When my son Harry was three years old, he was also one of these control children. The sight of a three-year-old facing a 4,300-calorie breakfast is every bit as ludicrous as it sounds. What did Harry do? He drank a glass of milk, took a bite of toast, threw the Rice Crispies onto the floor and that was pretty much it. Because every gram of food had to be measured in and measured out, the poor guys running the study then had to pick up every particle of puffed rice that was trodden into the floor. Anyway, to our collective surprise, when all the numbers were crunched, we found that the degree to which the receptor was dysfunctional could predict how much a child carrying that specific mutation would eat.[20] In other words, the MC4R does not act in binary fashion, as an on/off switch; rather it acts as a rheostat controlling appetite.

While measuring the actual amount of food eaten is important, understanding why we make particular food choices is less straightforward, and is also going to have critical implications for our understanding of obesity. Some of us love fatty foods in particular, others have a sweet tooth, while many others love high-fat AND high-sugar foods (desserts, anyone?). But what influences food choice? The taste, appearance, smell and texture of food are all important, but biology may also play an important role. In order to tackle this question, Sadaf devised two different experiments, this time to try to measure whether MC4R played a role in influencing food choice. She tested lean and obese individuals (as controls), and obese individuals carrying MC4R mutations. In the first experiment, she gave participants an all-you-can-eat buffet with three options of chicken korma (a mild curry with a sweet almond base). The three curries were the same, in look, smell and taste, but differed in fat content, which was manipulated to provide a 'Goldilocks' selection of 20 per cent (low), 40 per cent (medium) and 60 per cent (high) of the calories from fat. The participants were then asked to eat however much they wanted of all three. What happened was those carrying a mutation in MC4R ate almost twice the amount of high-fat curry than the lean individuals ate, and 65 per cent more than obese individuals without MC4R mutations.

In the second experiment, the same three groups were given Eton mess (a smashed-up Pavlova of strawberries, whipped cream and meringue). Again, there were three options from which to choose, this time differing in the amount of sugar present in the meringue, providing 8 per cent (low), 26 per cent (medium) and 54 per cent (high) of calorific content. Paradoxically, in contrast to the fat-choice experiment, individuals with a mutation in MC4R liked the high-sugar dessert less than their lean and obese counterparts and in fact ate significantly less of all three desserts compared to the other two groups. It turns out that people with a defective MC4R have an increased preference for high-fat food, but a decreased preference for sugary foods.[21] The fact that the MC4R pathway is not working may lead to them preferring high-fat food without realising it and therefore contributes to their weight problem. Thus, the melanocortin pathway not only allows for fine-tuning of the amount of food you might eat, but also influences your food preference.

NOT JUST US HUMANS

Typically, after the publication of a big research paper, you 'go on tour' on the conference circuit to tell your story, to network, get further collaborations, etc. It's a bit like being a rock star, but without the big hair (or in my case no hair), entourage, roadies, a tour bus or, truthfully, anyone really noticing. And so it was after we had published the story of the first MC4R patient in 1998. I spoke in San Diego, Paris, Taos (in New Mexico) and, more often than not, in far less exotic locales, such as the ageing Victorian seaside town of Bournemouth, on the south coast of England, where I was speaking at a meeting on an early spring day in 1999. I had just stepped off the stage after giving my talk, when a very well-presented lady approached me. I immediately clocked that she was far too well dressed to be an academic (we academics are a frumpy lot). '*Hmmmm . . . Pharmaceutical rep? Biotech? Press?*' I thought to myself. She handed me her card (academics don't carry cards either, so I had nothing to reciprocate with but my smile) and introduced herself:

'Hi, I'm Helen, I represent a . . .' At that exact same point I flipped the card around to have a look '. . . pig-breeding company.'

I did NOT expect that. I looked up to stare at her, 'You are a *farmer*?!'

'No!' she laughed and replied, 'but we do supply farmers.'

Anyway, Helen bought me a coffee, and it turned out that she had read our paper and had recognised certain characteristics in some of their pig breeds; naturally eats a lot, fast-growing and gets really large, has more fat but also has more muscle. Inspired by our findings, they investigated and found that these pigs, which are particularly prized for the quality of their back-bacon, carried mutations in the MC4R.[22] Helen told me, 'These pigs look like they are on steroids, but are not. They are as they are because of their genes. This means a lot to our farmers, who don't want to use growth supplements. So the role of the MC4R extends even into the agricultural industry.

But the importance of the melanocortin pathway in controlling appetitive behaviour and bodyweight goes beyond mammals. Mexican cavefish live in dark, isolated caves in north-eastern Mexico. They separated from their surface-dwelling cousins hundreds of thousands of years ago and have adapted to their environment in a number of different ways. For example, because they live in complete darkness, they gradually lost their eyes and pigmentation; and in a cave with little food, they became resistant to starvation. The cavefish can withstand months without food by storing massive amounts of fat and burning it more slowly. They also have evolved insatiable appetites so that when food does become available, swept in by floods perhaps once a year, the fish are able to eat without limit and store as much fat as they can to sustain them until the next feast. As it turns out, the root to this adaptation in feeding behaviour is a mutation in their MC4R gene.[23]

Tall, large humans with a penchant for high-fat chicken curry; organic, naturally fast-growing pigs producing artisan back bacon; and fat, binge-eating, blind cave fish – all because of mutations in the MC4R gene, leading to a defective MC4R protein that responds sub-optimally to melanocortin peptides.

WHERE YOU PUT YOUR FAT VS HOW MUCH FAT YOU HAVE

While all humans (all mammals in fact) share this melanocortin 'fuel sensor', we come in all different shapes and sizes. It is now becoming clear that this variation in body shape and weight has powerful genetic influences. Yet genetic disruption of the leptin–melanocortin pathway resulting in severe obesity remains a rare occurrence. The 'common' obesity that currently blights us is more likely to be 'polygenic' in origin ('poly' for many, genic for gene – so 'many-genes', this is in contrast to 'monogenic' or single-gene), with many subtle genetic variants, each in itself with an almost imperceptible effect, together having a cumulative measurable consequence. The problem with subtle and imperceptible effects, of course, is that it makes it very difficult indeed to track down the responsible genes, which frustrated the efforts of research into common obesity in the late 20th century. The only way to tackle this was to try and increase 'power'; meaning increasing the number of genes we could look at and the number of people we could do it in, by a LOT. Then at the turn of the millennium, rapidly evolving technological and computational developments meant that by using contemporary genetic approaches, we could now simultaneously assay millions of genetic variants in hundreds of thousands of people (relatively) cheaply and easily. These new genome-wide association studies (GWAS) revolutionised the study of complex diseases.

The first obesity GWAS was reported in 2007,[24] and in the intervening period since then many more have been published. Most of these have looked at BMI,[25] which, while imperfect, is an empirical and very easy to obtain proxy for how MUCH fat we carry. When I say empirical, I mean that it is a measure that does not rely on anyone's memory, or opinion. This is not (yet) true about what we eat or how much we eat, at least on a population basis (more about this later in the book). BMI can change over time of course, but at any moment in time, it does not lie and it is what it is. Other studies have looked at waist-to-hip ratio (WHR),[26] which is another easy-to-obtain and informative empirical measure. This is the ratio of your waist circumference to your hip circumference. If you look in the mirror, you will realise that what WHR informs us about is our body shape. Do you have a big tummy and a small bum? Do you have a large 'booty' but are skinny up top? Or are you simply the same size all over, like a sausage? This, ultimately, is about WHERE you put your fat.

While knowledge of actual mechanisms is still thin on the ground, a surprisingly cogent narrative has emerged from GWAS regarding the genetic architecture of common obesity.[27] I have attempted to summarise this below and in figure 7 following:

a) WHERE you put your fat (WHR) has very little (genetically at least) to do with HOW MUCH fat you have (BMI);

b) your WHR is influenced by genes that are primarily expressed in fat and play a role in fat biology;

c) your BMI is influenced by genes primarily expressed in the brain. Amongst these are genes for many components of the melanocortin pathway, including POMC and MC4R, which regulate food intake.

To clarify, GWAS suggests that **where** you put your fat has to do with **fat biology,** whereas **how much** fat you have has to do with your **brain** and your **feeding behaviour.** To be crystal clear, what GWAS look at are not disruptive loss-of-function mutations that cause severe obesity, like those we've discussed for much of this chapter. Rather, they look at subtle variations in genes that are found in all of us. Some of the variants are associated with being slightly heavier, which have been labelled as 'risk variants'; while others are associated with being lean and have been labelled as 'protective variants'. However, this is only because we are looking at the data through the prism of a modern obesity epidemic. Whereas in the past, when there was not enough food and we were all trying to stave off starvation, the labels might easily be reversed!

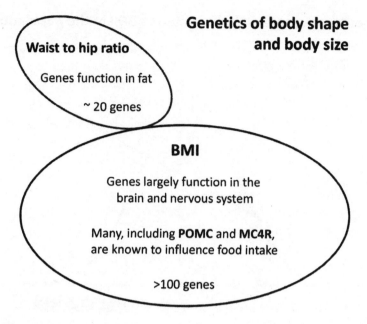

FIGURE 7

In fact, one can actually create a 'risk score' for our likelihood of becoming obese.[28] Consider each genetic variant having a possible score of 2 (homozygous or possessing 2 copies of the risk variant), 1 (heterozygous or possessing 1 copy of the risk and 1 copy of the protective variant) or 0 (no risk variants but 2 copies of the protective variant). As there are around 100 genes linked to BMI, that is a notional maximum risk score of 200 (100 x 2) and a minimum of 0. But biology being what it is, the reality is the risk scores within a population will fit a 'bell curve' (see figure), otherwise known as a 'normal distribution'. What this means is most of us will have a risk score that sits in a relatively narrow range around an average of 100, while a few of us will have very low or very high risk scores. However, when plotted against a large enough population, what we observe is the higher your obesity risk score, the higher your BMI is likely to be (the diagonal line in the figure). What we have here is an illustration of polygenics influencing a complex

Obesity risk score directly related to BMI in the population

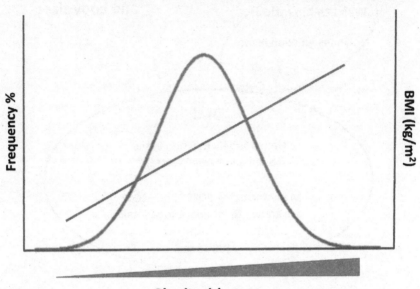

FIGURE 8

trait. In spite of what is very often reported in the media, there is no single 'fat gene' when it comes to common obesity. Rather, we all have our own personal mix of risk vs protective variants that places us on the normal distribution of bodyweight. What the data tells us is that having more 'risk' variants of some of these genes influences our brain, making it slightly less sensitive to hormones from the fat and gut; other variants modulate the rewarding feeling we get from food; and yet others might influence how neurons communicate with each other. The sum effect is that people with a higher risk score simply feel a little more hungry all of the time, which makes it more difficult for them to say 'no', meaning they are likely to eat more, and are hence more likely to become obese. And critically, when it is more difficult to say 'no', it is also far more challenging to lose weight once you become obese.

It is interesting to note that, to date, there are no genes that have been convincingly linked to metabolism and energy expenditure. This does not mean that differences in metabolism don't influence BMI. There are indeed people who can eat more than others, yet not become obese. While food intake data can be collected on a large scale using food diaries and questionnaires (albeit imperfectly), energy expenditure is just a far more complex characteristic to measure accurately at a population level (I go into this in detail in Chapter 12).

IT'S ALL IN OUR HEAD

There is still the strongly held belief in many quarters that we are in full 'executive control' of our own eating behaviour; that the environment is responsible for our shape and size, and that our genes, our 'nature', has minimal, if any, effect. However, it is crucial to remember that the drive to consume food is one of the most primitive of instincts to promote survival. It has been shaped by many millions of years of evolution and has provided living creatures with powerful and redundant mechanisms to adapt and respond to times of nutrient scarcity. Thus, I would argue that to be overweight in our current environment is indeed the natural – highly evolved, even – response. In this chapter, I have shown that this response is due, in large part, to genes that function within our brain. Obesity is, in fact, 'all in the head'.

The main issue is that this environment, in which energy-dense foods and stimulatory food cues are ubiquitous, coupled with concurrent changes in lifestyle, is in dissonance with the millennia of austere surroundings to which we have adapted. This has consequently pushed obesity to become the serious problem it is today. I am fully aware that without this 'obesogenic' environment, most of us would not be overweight or obese; but to deny the central role that our genes have played in our response to this environment is unhelpful as we strive to tackle one of the greatest public health challenges of the 21st century.

CHAPTER 3

All calories are equal, but some are more equal than others

My research lab is based at Addenbrooke's Hospital on the Cambridge Biomedical Campus, located three miles south of Cambridge town centre – what I call 'Disneyland', because all of the old buildings make it seem like a theme park. It is one of the largest biomedical campuses in Europe; a major tertiary medical centre with world-leading experts in most diseases; and it contains many international leading research institutes, including the famous Medical Research Council Laboratory of Molecular Biology (MRC LMB). During the past fifty years, the MRC LMB's scientists have received twelve Nobel prizes, most recently in 2018 – twelve from just one building . . . incredible. All in all, more than 10,000 people work on the biomedical campus. If you include the thousands of out- and inpatients that are at the hospital on any given day, that adds up to nearly 15,000 people. Given that the population of Cambridge is around 125,000, that is more than 10 per cent of the populace that works or visits the biomedical campus every day.

The campus is far enough away from the town centre that everyone there is, in effect, a captive audience. The amenities available at the hospital reflect this: there is a bank, a hairdresser, a clothing and gift shop, a newsagent, a branch of a city law firm (for divorces and real estate, apparently), four espresso coffee bars, and food. Lots of food. The food court is populated with well-known international brands, including a burger joint whose name, shall we say, references the monarchy. Just recently, a major supermarket chain joined the fray and opened an 'express' store; one of these places that sells primarily convenience food and drink. I was there one day, getting a sandwich for lunch, with what appeared to be everyone else in the hospital, and happened to overhear a conversation between two ladies.

'My diet only allows me 400 calories for lunch . . .'

'How about this one? Wild salmon and cucumber on soft oatmeal. It says it is only 386 calories.'

'No, I'll take the prawn sandwich. 376 calories it says . . . that means I can have an extra cookie at tea-time.'

That day, I lived life on the edge and splashed out an entire 459 calories on a Coronation Chicken sandwich, 277 calories on a bag of Flame Grilled Steak and Onion Crisps, less than one calorie on a diet soda, and I skipped the cookie at tea-time. Where it used to be hidden in some microscopic unreadable font at the back of the pack, the calorie count of everything is now placed front and centre. Even if I had chosen the burger option for lunch (I don't tell my wife when I do), the number of calories for each item is right there on the menu board (large cheeseburger 760 calories . . . and you really don't want to know how many calories there are in the 'meal' option, which includes large fries and soda (north of 1,400 calories if you plump for the full sugar beverage!)). The calorie counts are there, ostensibly, to empower consumers. To allow people to make informed choices. To enable the two calorie-counting ladies, whose conversation I eavesdropped on, to achieve a sub-400 calorie lunch.

In reality however, how useful is it to know how many calories there are in a given item of food? If something has more calories, does that mean it is bad for you? Are foods with fewer calories automatically better for you? Are all calories equal? That's what I'd like to focus on in this chapter.

CALORIE WITH A BIG 'C' OR A SMALL 'c'?

First of all, what exactly is a calorie? A calorie is a unit of energy, that much most of us will know. It is, for those of you who prefer to work in metric measures, equivalent to 4.184 joules, but that is not particularly helpful in making things any clearer. Oddly, it also matters if we are talking about a calorie with a big 'C' or a small 'c'. 'Pardon?' I hear you say, 'Have we suddenly wandered on to the set of *Sesame Street*?' A calorie (small 'c') is the amount of energy it takes to raise the temperature of 1 gram of water (which is equivalent to 1 millilitre (ml) of water at sea-level) by 1°C, whereas a Calorie (big 'C') is the amount of energy it takes to raise the temperature of 1 kilogram (or 1 litre at sea-level) of water by 1°C. There are 1,000 mls in a litre, so a big 'C' Calorie is also known as a kilocalorie (or a Kcal). The confusing thing is that the calories that we ALL refer to, and that appear on the menu boards and food packages are actually Kcals, or a Calorie with a big 'C'. I am presuming that 'calorie' is just a whole lot easier to say than kilocalorie, or Kcal, or big 'C' Calorie, so it has stuck! Be that as it may, let's just be clear that whenever I refer to a calorie in the rest of this book, I am referring to Kcals.

CALORIC AVAILABILITY

The original and still most accurate method of determining the caloric content of food is with a 'bomb calorimeter'. It is as violent and unsophisticated as the name suggests. In effect, you put an item of food into a sealed container, the eponymous 'bomb', and then you burn everything to an absolute crisp, literally carbonising the food. Because the 'bomb' is sealed, nothing escapes, and all of the heat given off during the burning process is captured by a surrounding water jacket. The resulting increase in water temperature in the jacket is then used to calculate the amount of energy or calories contained within the item of food, which is released during the combustion process. And just in case you were wondering, food that is too wet to be burnt, like soup or milk or fruit for instance, is desiccated first. As water contains no calories, removing it doesn't impact the calorie count. Since a calorie (Kcal) is a unit of energy, equivalent to 4,184 joules or 4.184 kilojoules, then all calories are clearly equal.

The inside of a bomb calorimeter, however, is an extreme environment, and is designed as such to ensure that every single calorie is accounted for. The biological process of food digestion within a living being is a little gentler. Apart from a bit of chewing at the very beginning, digestion is, by and large, a series of chemical reactions, accelerated by biological catalysts called enzymes. Don't get me wrong, it is still quite a harsh process; you wouldn't want to stick your hand into your stomach juices for instance, as it bears a strong resemblance to battery acid – but it isn't anything like a bonfire. As a result, depending on its structure and content, how it has been processed, as well as who or what is eating and performing the actual digestion, each item of food will have a different caloric availability. This is a critically important concept to grasp. *Caloric availability is the amount of calories that can actually be extracted during the digestion process, as opposed to the total number of calories that are locked up in the food.*

Let me give you a few examples. The simplest item of food you can probably consume is sugar. The term 'sugar' encompasses many different compounds: glucose, fructose, lactose, galactose, sucrose … most compounds ending in '-ose' essentially. The powdered and granulated form that is most commonly used and available in shops is sucrose, which is one molecule each of glucose and fructose joined together. Sucrose is therefore a 'disaccharide' as opposed to either glucose or fructose, which are 'monosaccharides'.

If you ate 100 calories of sugar, the digestion process just needs to split sucrose into its constituent parts, and you would extract well over 95 calories. Glucose is, after all, our basic unit of fuel. What happens, however, if we eat 100 calories of sweetcorn or 'corn-on-the-cob'? We might have chewed it and swallowed it, but, if we happened to peek down as we were sat on the porcelain throne the next day, it would be quite obvious that our digestive system would only have managed to extract a fraction of the total calories that were on offer. It is clear we would have absorbed nowhere near the 100 calories of energy in the corn. This is, in fact, such a well-known phenomenon that sweetcorn is the primary tool used to determine 'bowel transit time', which is the length of time it takes for food to travel through the digestive tract, from mouth to colon, and is used as a marker of bowel health. Consider, though, if the same amount of sweetcorn had instead been desiccated, ground into corn meal, mixed with some water and then made into corn tortillas. All of a sudden, a far larger fraction of the 100 calories tied up in those yellow kernels is accessible by the body. Yet, if you go to the store and buy equivalent amounts of sugar, sweetcorn or corn tortillas, the nutritional information at the back of all three packages would still say 100 calories.

Another classic example is celery. Celery is famously thought to have 'negative calories', whereby the amount of energy required to digest it outstrips the amount of extractable calories. This is apocryphal and not true.[1] That being said, the amount of calories available to the human digestive system from a single medium-sized stick of raw celery is a minuscule six calories, which is positive energy, but only just barely. The reason for this is that much of its caloric content, as is the case with the sweetcorn kernels, is bound up in cellulose, a fibre that humans just can't digest. If you cook the same amount of celery, however, in a stew or soup or gumbo for instance, you begin to break down the cellulose, and as a consequence more than quadruple the amount of available energy to nearly 30 calories. Think about it, a more than four-fold difference in caloric availability in exactly the same food item depending on how it has been prepared or processed. Celery is probably the most extreme example. But while the actual numbers will differ, the same principle holds true for many other vegetables, like carrots, cabbage, broccoli, beans, etc.

How about foods that have no cellulose? Meat, for instance? Well, 100 grams of skinless and boneless raw chicken breast has 114 available calories, whereas when cooked (roasted), its caloric availability increases to 165 per 100 grams. These and countless other caloric measurements can be found on the US Department of Agriculture (USDA) Food Composition Database.[2] OK, we don't (and shouldn't) eat raw chicken, so this is possibly not the most relevant of examples. How about beef instead? We can eat 400 calories of beef as a steak that has been cooked rare or even 'blue', which is pretty much raw, except for a quick searing of the outer layer to kill off any bugs. In contrast, you can take that same piece of beef, mince it, stew it as a meat sauce for a couple of hours, layer it into a lasagne and cook it for a further couple of hours, freeze it for a rainy day, take it out of the freezer on a rainy day and heat it in the oven for an additional hour, before a fork-full of lasagne eventually meets your lips. Contrast the 2–6 minutes it takes to grill a steak to the five hours of cooking it takes to produce a lasagne. If the comparison between the raw and cooked chicken is anything to go by, our digestive tract is going to be able to extract a lot more calories from a piece of beef when it has been lent a helping hand by 5 hours of pretty intensive heat treatment.

On top of food preparation, processing and cooking, one has to consider how much energy it takes to break down the individual components of protein, carbs and fat. What happens once these macronutrients have been chewed in our mouth, acid-treated in our stomach and entered our small intestine? Protein takes the most energy and the longest time to digest, with nearly 30 per cent of the total calories eaten in protein required to digest it from the long chains they exist as in intact food, to individual amino acids.[3] This means that for every 100 calories of lean beef or chicken or other meat you eat, it would cost you 30 calories to digest it, leaving you with around 70 calories. But as I've discussed, how the meat has been processed and cooked will significantly influence this number. Carbohydrates take anywhere from 5–10 per cent of consumed calories to digest, depending on whether we're talking about complex starches, which would cost more, or simple sugars which would cost less. Finally, fat is the most efficient of our fuels, requiring only around 3 per cent of consumed calories to digest.

The problem is that the measurement of caloric availability in a real-world scenario is not trivial. Accurate figures for the vast majority of food items are simply not available, and there is the added complexity that caloric availability is likely to differ (very subtly, but there will be differences) between individuals. But it isn't entirely impossible and we really need to do better. For one thing, we could and should find a way of factoring in the different calorie costs for digesting protein, carbs and fat. There are obviously issues to address, such as what methods of preparation should be included in making the calculation? You can imagine the back of a packet of beef, chicken or pork going on and on for ever, encompassing a multitude of different recipes, which is clearly also not the solution. Don't get me wrong, I love both steak and lasagne, as well as cooking fast on a grill and slow in the oven. My point is that the current displaying of caloric content expressly as a health or weight-loss tool is not fully fit for purpose. It is true that calorie labels added to menus or put next to food in restaurants, coffee shops and cafeterias, can reduce calories purchased by about 8 per cent per meal.[4] So calorie information at point of purchase does seem to give people pause for thought, and appears to influence decisions. However, calorie counting in a diet-plan, like those ladies trying to stick to 400 calories for lunch, simply makes no sense without taking into account, or at least even acknowledging, caloric availability.

WHEN YOU EAT THE CALORIES MATTER

The 2017 Nobel Prize in Medicine and Physiology went to three scientists: Jeffrey C. Hall, Michael Rosbash and Michael W. Young, for their work on understanding the regulation of the body-clock, or circadian rhythm.[5] The original work was done on the humble fruit fly, the tiny ones that hang about when your bananas start to go brown. You might think that there is nothing much in common between flies and humans, and clearly we are very different creatures. Compared to humans, for instance, flies have fewer genes (14,000 vs 25,000 in humans). That being said, 14,000 is still more than half the number of human genes, and 60 per cent of our genes actually have a fruit-fly equivalent.

The best way of understanding the function of a gene is to disrupt it and to see what happens. In fact, much of what we know about human biology has come from studying rare (and sometimes not so rare), naturally occurring, catastrophic disruption of genes, so-called 'experiments of nature'; the children with the mutations in their leptin or MC4R genes are cases in point. However, engineering a genetic disruption in humans is not possible (for obvious moral and ethical reasons) and remains time-consuming and labour-intensive in mice. However, it is relatively cheap and straightforward to mutate a fly gene. This, coupled with their small size, short lifecycle and high reproductive rate, has led the fruit fly to become a very widely used genetic tool.

In 1984, Jeffrey and the two Michaels isolated a gene that controls the normal daily biological rhythm of the fruit fly.[6] They subsequently went on to identify other components of this clock.

We now know that biological clocks exist not only in flies, but in all plants and organisms, including in us humans.

Because all life on earth has had to adapt to our planet's rotation, internal biological clocks have evolved, allowing plants and organisms to synchronise their biological rhythms to the day/night cycle. Humans, for instance, are diurnal creatures, meaning we are awake in the day and asleep at night. Because our clock regulates critical functions such as behaviour, hormone levels, sleep, body temperature and metabolism, we are consequently more alert, better coordinated and have faster reaction times during the day. Even wounds received during the day heal faster than if you are wounded at night![7] Nocturnal creatures, such as bats or mice, will of course have their clocks reversed, and thus be awake at night instead. Those of you who have experienced 'jetlag' will know what it feels like not to be synchronised to the time of day; that inevitable haze of fog that descends at the most inopportune of times, such as in the middle of a meeting where you really need to concentrate, or suddenly feeling the desperate need for your bed at 3 p.m. in the afternoon. Many thousands of years ago on the Serengeti, having our biological clock correctly synchronised to the time of day was critical, as it ensured that we were in the optimum physical and mental condition at the appropriate time to successfully hunt and forage for food, while at the same avoiding becoming food. Part of the adaptation that allowed us to be more physically responsive in the daytime is that our metabolism, the rate at which we burn and use fuel, is higher during the day then at night. What this means is that whether the calories we eat are more likely to be burnt or stored depends on the time of day they were consumed. Put another way, *when* we eat during the day really does matter.

'Eat breakfast like a king, lunch like a prince and dinner like a pauper' is an old adage in many cultures. The Chinese version of this is a rhyme I learnt as a child; 早餐要吃好 *(zao can yao chi hao)*, 午餐要吃饱 *(wu can yao chi bao)*, 晚餐要吃少 *(wan can yao chi shao)*, which translates to a less poetic 'Eat well for breakfast, eat till you're full for lunch, and eat less for dinner'. For the vast majority of human existence, we, of course, had no electricity. While candles have been around for a long time, with some archaeological evidence dating them back to 5000 BC, they remained a luxury for most throughout history. Life therefore revolved around the rising and setting sun and people went to bed when it got dark. This meant that most of the cooking and eating happened during the day. The term 'dinner' used to refer to the main, and largest, meal of the day, which for much of history was around midday. In the UK, the midday meal served to primary and secondary school students is still referred to as 'school dinner'.

The concept of the large evening meal, now called dinner in most of the English-speaking world, is thus really quite modern. But is eating your main meal in the evening, and therefore going against the 'old-wives' tales' from many different cultures, actually bad for you? Some evidence has begun to emerge that appears to support this. In one study, 420 participants on a 20-week weight-loss programme were divided into groups according to the time when they had lunch, which was, in this situation, their main daily meal. Intriguingly, despite no difference in amount of food eaten or its dietary composition, those who ate later in the day lost less weight and at a slower rate than compared to those who ate earlier.[8] In another experiment, overweight women were placed on identical diets, but were different in the proportion of calories distributed between breakfast and dinner. The women eating more at breakfast ended up losing 9 per cent more weight than those eating more at dinner.[9]

Wow, this data does seem quite damning about the modern cultural phenomenon of dinner in the evening being our main meal. But there are some important caveats to consider. For one thing, these studies were focussed on people actively trying to lose weight, all eating the same amount of food and differing only in the time of day they were eating. In other words, these are good examples of actual 'experiments', where there was only one controllable variable being examined. The differences that were picked up, which were relatively subtle, were seen in the amount of weight and the rate at which it was lost.

How about the effects of eating at different times of the day in people not actively on a diet? The data here is less clear. There is some evidence that eating after 8 p.m. in the evening is associated with increased BMI,[10] but equally there are many studies that don't show this. The problem is that unlike the weight-loss experiments above, these are not 'experiments' *per se*, but are 'observational studies'. Observational studies are where researchers observe a group or population in order to draw inferences, but where key variables, such as in this case how much is being eaten and when, are not controllable. These studies are still hugely important, but are inherently noisy. What we can infer, however, is that even if the timing of our meals does have a significant influence on our bodyweight, the effects are likely to be subtle and only observable at a population level. At any rate, because the vast majority of us work in the day, and really only have time to have our main meal in the evening, the pragmatic reality is that dinner will be an evening meal for the foreseeable future. That being said, if one were trying to reduce the amount of calories consumed in an effort to lose weight, cutting a larger proportion of those calories from the evening meal, as opposed to breakfast or lunch, might be a sensible decision to make.

WHERE DO THE SPARE CALORIES GO?

So once the food we've eaten is chewed; acid-treated; enzymatically digested into sugar, amino acids and fatty acids within our small intestines; and then absorbed into our bloodstream, where do all of the nutrients go to? Obviously the first priority is that they are instantly put to work to fuel the running of our body. Anything we don't use immediately, however, which is going to be the case for most of the calories we consume, we would then need a strategy to store for future use. We are not hummingbirds after all – unlike them, we do not need to constantly eat in order to survive.

Any fat we eat that we don't use immediately will naturally go into our fat stores. Excess protein is used to provide your body with energy, and if you are weightlifting is put into muscle. However, the reality is that you can't store extra amino acids or protein for later use. Anything not immediately used is actually turned into fat. So if you consume too many calories in an effort to increase your protein intake you will gain weight. As for spare glucose, around 25g, or about 100 calories, circulates in the blood. A larger amount is converted into glycogen. Skeletal muscles store about 400g of glycogen and the liver stores about 90–110g. All of this equates to about 2,000 calories of carbohydrates that your body is capable of storing, which is probably a couple of days' worth. Glycogen is an energy reserve that can be mobilised quickly to meet a sudden need for glucose. The reason we 'carbo-load' the night before the big race is to top up the glycogen stores in the muscle and liver, so that we can use it as an easily available source of glucose while we are long-distance running, or cycling, or swimming, or hiking. Glycogen, however, while easily accessible, is not a very efficient way of storing energy. The problem is, to form 1 gram of glycogen, you need 3 grams of water, which means that there will always be an upper limit of around 500 grams of glycogen you can store, as it retains so much water. Contrast this to fat, which contains no water at all, and is therefore energetically very dense. An average-size adult of healthy weight has between 10 and 20 kilograms of fat stores, which equates to about 90,000–180,000 calories! Thus, all of the spare glucose not stored as glycogen is converted into fat. So in actuality, when we ask the question 'where do the spare calories go?' the answer is almost entirely into fat.

WHAT IS FAT?

'Fat' is a term, used pejoratively or not, depending on intent and tone, to describe someone on the larger side. We also use it as a noun to refer to the excess tissue that is carried by all of us, with some carrying more than others. The scientific term for the adjective 'fat' is of course either overweight or obese, depending on how large someone is. The scientific term for fat, the noun, is 'adipose tissue', a loose connective tissue formed largely of adipocytes, which are the individual fat cells. Each adipocyte is like an empty balloon, designed to store excess energy coming from dietary fat, protein or carbohydrates. As spare energy is converted into lipids, they enter the adipocyte and form a large single lipid droplet, taking up most of the volume of the cell, continuing to grow and grow, eventually expanding the adipocyte like a balloon. When you gain weight, while some new adipocytes do form, the increase in fat mass is largely a function of expanding balloon-like adipocytes filling with lipids. Conversely, in weight loss, you do not lose your fat cells; rather, as you use up the excess lipids, your adipocytes shrink. While carbohydrates are more easily mobilised and are, as a result, often used first, the body runs mainly on fat, which typically provides more than half of the body's energy needs. After all, a gram of carbohydrate releases 4 calories, the same as for protein, whereas a gram of fat when fully metabolised releases 9 calories.

For the longest time, people had thought of fat as passive and largely biologically inert. It provides cushioning – just imagine your derrière without a little bit of padding as you sit down . . . doesn't sound too comfortable; it provides insulation; and it is there as our primary long-term energy store. However, because how much fat we carry is how long we would last without food, it is critical that our brain knows this piece of information. Once the adipocyte hormone leptin was discovered,[11] fat suddenly joined the pantheon of other hormone-producing organs, otherwise known as 'endocrine' organs. Leptin circulates in the blood to reflect fat mass and is sensed by the brain; but as it turns out, was just the first of many hormones secreted by fat to be discovered. Because the amount of fat is important to the functioning of many biological functions, such as reproduction and our immune system, our fat keeps in communication with the brain and other organs through the secretion of a whole repertoire of different hormones.[12]

IT'S NOT JUST HOW MUCH YOU HAVE, BUT WHERE YOU PUT IT

Why is being obese unhealthy?

'It's because you are carrying too much fat', I hear many of you say. That statement may be a description of the problem, but doesn't explain it.

OK, so WHY is carrying too much fat bad for you?

This has actually turned out to be a surprisingly complex question, which, while much progress has been made in recent years, we in the field are still not completely able to answer. However, some key ideas have emerged that appear to address a significant portion of the question, although the devil is always in the detail.

The most visibly obvious reason that carrying too much fat is bad for you is a purely mechanical one; that is, the battle against gravity. Being too heavy can clearly slow you down, making you physically less active, which means you lose muscle mass, leading to a vicious downward cycle. Being obese also puts you at risk of sleep apnoea, a disorder in which one's airway becomes obstructed while asleep; causing, in its most benign form, loud snoring, and a complete cessation of breathing, cardiac arrhythmias and low blood oxygen levels at its worst. Excess weight also takes its toll on joints, with obesity linked to increased risk of osteoarthritis, particularly of the knee, compared to those in a healthy weight range. However, it is rarely obesity itself that ends up killing us. Rather it is the accompanying host of diseases that are closely linked to obesity, such as type 2 diabetes, cardiovascular disease, high blood pressure and certain cancers, which serve to amplify and exacerbate the problem.

But why does carrying too much fat lead to these comorbidities? The answers to this question are complex and the subject of furious ongoing and cutting-edge research. There are three broad schools of thought that have emerged, and they are not mutually exclusive of each other.

The first is the concept of lipotoxicity,[13] which quite literally means to be poisoned by fat. Fat (the noun) gets a bad rap, but at the end of the day, it is the job of adipose tissue to safely store excess lipids and fatty acids for later use. But what happens if your fat stores become 'full'? As I mentioned previously, adipocytes expand like a balloon to store lipids. They cannot, however, expand indefinitely, and at some point will reach capacity. An adipocyte will not pop like a balloon (here the analogy ends), but no more lipids will be able to be taken up. Lipids that can't be stored in fat have to go somewhere else, and end up in tissues that are not designed to safely store them in large amounts, such as your muscles and your liver. Because the lipids are not supposed to be there, they begin to affect the function of these tissues and organs. For example, because of the huge amount of physical work they undertake, most of the glucose in the blood is absorbed by your muscles, and it is consequently the biggest store of glycogen in the body. After a meal, blood glucose levels rise, which triggers a sharp rise in the levels of insulin produced by the pancreas. Your muscles respond to this rise in insulin by taking up glucose and converting it to glycogen. However, the presence of large amounts of lipids interferes with this process, leading the muscles to become 'insulin resistant'. This means that for every unit of insulin, less glucose is taken up by the muscles. This is not good because humans are evolved to function optimally within quite a small window of glucose concentration (4–7 millimolar). To overcome this, your pancreas begins to work harder to produce more insulin. Every organ in the body is designed to function at a particular rate for a certain length of time, very much like a car is designed to travel for a certain distance, with the engine working within a particular window of effort. Having your pancreas working harder is like having the engine in your car work harder than it was designed to do, meaning that your car will not travel as far. In some susceptible individuals, once they become insulin resistant, their pancreas simply can't cope with the increased rate of work and begins to slow down, meaning that blood glucose levels cannot be maintained within the normal healthy range, and the person becomes diabetic. This type of diabetes is known as type 2 diabetes. In contrast, type 1 diabetes is where your immune system attacks and destroys the pancreatic cells that produce insulin, which is a different and more acute condition, and requires daily injections of insulin in order to treat it.

The second concept is that it isn't just too much fat that can cause problems, but that where you put the fat actually influences the severity of the problem. Where you put your fat largely determines your body-shape and, as I discussed in Chapter 2, is powerfully genetically influenced. Are you big in the middle, but have relatively skinny arms and legs, so-called 'apple' shaped? Do you perhaps have a larger bum and legs, with a smaller top, so-called 'pear' shaped? Or are you large all over?

An apple-shaped person is typically, although not exclusively, male, and has accumulated a lot of fat around their organs. This type of fat is also known as visceral fat, and tends to result in a large but tight belly, the stereotypical 'beer-belly'. This contrasts with the fat that sits just under the skin, which is known as sub-cutaneous (subcut) fat. We are obviously entirely covered in skin, so subcut fat can accumulate pretty much anywhere.

A pear-shaped individual is typically, although not exclusively, female, and carries fat primarily around the bum and legs. Subcut fat can also sit under the arms, allowing you to measure its 'wobble factor'. Lift up one of your arms as if you were about to admire your biceps; now without tensing up, give the flesh under your arm a gentle push. Does it move back and forth just once, or does it swing multiple times (this is the wobble factor) like a pendulum? Subcut fat also accumulates around the belly of both males and females, but because it sits under the skin, is 'flabbier' or more 'wobbly' than a beer-belly. I am not using any of these terms pejoratively and am not intending to offend; I am hoping these adjectives are descriptive enough so you can calculate the 'wobble factor' of your arms, or look down at your own (or your loved one's) belly and figure out what kind of fat (if you are fat) you are carrying more of. I can report for instance (and my wife will testify to this), that my arms have little to no wobble factor, whereas, reflecting my BMI of 26, my belly is larger than it should be, and because it is wobbly, is likely to be the result of an accumulation of excess subcut fat. The other place where I tend to accumulate subcut fat is around my cheeks . . . kind of like squirrel pouches, which my wife always reminds me about. I have a very spherical head; in fact my face is so round, you could probably use it to calculate a pretty close approximation of π (pi). What are wives for, after all, if not to inject a bit of reality into your day?

While you can do something about how MUCH fat you are carrying, you actually have next to no control over WHERE you put your fat. This is almost entirely down to your genes and your hormones (which are influenced by your genes of course, but also by how old you are). So why should you care about where your fat goes? That is because visceral fat in particular is linked to a higher risk of insulin resistance and diabetes, as well as an increased risk of strokes, heart disease and some cancers. It is, by far, worse for your health than fat anywhere else in your body. Because men tend to carry more visceral fat then women, they in turn have a higher risk of developing heart disease and other metabolic problems. The question is why? Is it a simple case of geography, where since visceral fat sits closer to our organs, it can cause more damage? That certainly could play a role, as visceral fat drains directly into the portal vein of the liver, probably not doing it a world of good.

However, studies performed in mice indicate a more complex picture. Scientists did an experiment where they transplanted visceral fat from around the organs to the backside of the mouse; it's like they gave the mouse a 'booty'. They then did the reciprocal experiment, where subcut fat was transferred to the viscera of mice.[14] What they found was that it didn't matter where either type of fat was sitting. Visceral fat remained unhealthy wherever it was, and moving subcut fat near the organs did not result in any metabolic harm. In other words, visceral fat is harmful not because of where it is, but because of what it is. I mentioned previously that fat is an endocrine organ that secretes hormones. Well, we now know that subcut fat and visceral fat are different tissues. While both are still formed from adipocytes and store lipids, visceral fat appears more dynamic. It is more responsive to certain hormones, contains more immune cells (see below), is metabolically more active and, critically, secretes a different repertoire of hormones compared to subcut fat. The link between visceral fat and metabolic and heart disease is down to a mix of these factors. We still don't have all of the answers though, and this is one of the hottest areas of metabolic science, with new findings emerging every day. Those of you now looking down at your rather large and unflabby but tight belly, it is not all doom and gloom. Evolutionarily, it appears that we have visceral fat because it generates a massive supply of energy from fatty acids when it is desperately needed, far more quickly than it can be mobilised and released from subcut fat. Thus, visceral fat is designed to be more responsive to lifestyle changes, such as improving your diet and increasing physical activity, as compared to subcut fat.

The third and final concept is that obesity appears to be a state of chronic inflammation.[15] Let's return to the analogy of an adipocyte being like balloon, in which there is a huge difference in size at both extremes, either empty or completely filled with lipids. When completely full of lipids, as would be the case in obesity, the adipocytes under a microscope almost look to be straining at the seams. In fact, the extreme stretching of the adipocyte almost seems to our body like damage and causes a mild inflammatory response, so much so that immune cells that normally respond to damaged tissue begin to infiltrate the fat of many obese people. Immune cells will infiltrate subcut fat as well, but appear to be more drawn to visceral fat. These immune cells secrete a large repertoire of factors that signal to other tissues and organs, in some cases causing insulin resistance. Once again, though, this is another area of metabolic research in which we don't have all of the answers.

Thus, while obese people undoubtedly face mechanical difficulties, it is the link between obesity and a whole host of associated, nasty diseases that ends up causing the real damage and putting severe pressure on our health-care systems. But I hope I've convinced you that obese people are going to respond in different ways to the excess calories that they are consuming, particularly in where they end up being stored.

THE SIZE OF YOUR 'BATH' MATTERS

Let us return to the concept of lipotoxicity, or being poisoned by lipids. This occurs when our fat cells have reached their maximal capacity, forcing excess lipids into tissues that are not designed to store them, thus driving, amongst other metabolic problems, insulin resistance, and for those who are susceptible, eventually leading to type 2 diabetes.

But hold on a minute. What exactly do we mean by 'maximal capacity'? Is this upper limit of fat storage universal? Do everyone's adipocytes expand to exactly the same maximum volume before lipids begin leaching into other tissues? Or is there natural variation in our ability to store fat?

In a large seminal study led by members of our institute, but conducted in collaboration with many others in the UK, it was found that there are indeed genetic influences on our ability to store fat.[16] Critically, the study also showed that the smaller a person's capacity to store fat, the more likely they are to become insulin resistant and eventually type 2 diabetic. Stephen O'Rahilly (recently made a knight of the realm; we now have our lab meetings at a round table), our moustachioed institute director and one of the senior authors on the study, gives an apt, if colourful, analogy that I feel compelled to share here.

This is the story of a bathroom with a carpeted floor.

OK, before I even begin, I already hear the question: *Who in their right mind carpets their bathroom?* Hold your questions till the end, please!

This is the story of a bathroom with a carpeted floor. In it stands an old-fashioned enamelled cast-iron bath. It has, over time, lost the plug for its plug-hole, so that when you begin to fill the bath, the water runs out down the drain. But eventually, with enough water going in, the bath begins to fill. Consider this bath analogous to our ability to store fat, with the water representing lipids, and if the bath overflows and wets the carpet, this then represents lipotoxicity (we all knew there was a reason for the carpet). In this scenario, there are two ways of preventing water overflowing (lipotoxicity): either you reduce the amount of water going in to the bath (this is reducing food intake), or you increase the size of the plug-hole to allow more water to safely run down the drain (this is increasing energy expenditure or physical activity). At some point, you will reach a safe equilibrium of the right amount of water flowing in and safely out the bath, without any overflow to wet the carpet. This is now someone eating and exercising appropriately, and therefore carrying a safe amount of fat.

Let us now tweak this scenario. What happens if we keep everything the same, except we make the bath smaller? Immediately you see that this reduces the amount of water (lipids) that can be safely held in the bath (fat storage capacity) before it overflows and wets the carpet (lipotoxicity). The converse would then happen if we increased the size of the bath. We would be able to store a lot more lipids before we were forced into lipotoxicity.

Here is the important message to take away from the bathroom and its damp carpet. All of us have 'baths' of different sizes, meaning we all have different fat-storage capacities. If we surpass our own personal fat-carrying capacity, we will tilt into metabolic disease. However, because of the natural variation in this capacity, some of us can carry more weight than others before becoming ill, whereas about 15 per cent of type 2 diabetics, for example, are not overweight at all, so are likely to have really small fat carrying capacities. I was in New Zealand a little while back to visit collaborators, and heard a talk comparing the incidence of type 2 diabetes in the local Polynesian population to the incidence of disease in the large immigrant population of South Asian Indians. The Polynesians, who are a famously large people, have to get to quite a high BMI before becoming diabetic. Whereas the immigrant population of Indians weighed, on average, substantially less than the Polynesians, yet had similar levels of type 2 diabetes.[17] The size of your 'bath' really matters.

Incidentally, this is why undergoing liposuction is one of the dumbest things you could do to try and lose weight and look better. You may end up having a more sculpted tummy or arms or bottom or thighs, but because you are actually removing fat cells, rather than the excess lipids within the cells, you are actually reducing the size of your 'bath'. So you may end up looking better, but you will actually end up more ill, with a far greater chance of type 2 diabetes, because you now have less safe fat-storage capacity. Remember, you want to reduce the size of your fat cells, but not reduce the number.

INCIDENTAL VIRTUOUS FOODS

We were talking about celery at the beginning of this chapter, and the myth that it has negative calories. Let's take a sojourn from fat storage for a minute and revisit that most fibrous of vegetables. While there are no foods with actual negative calories, some healthy foods, celery included, have been shown to have an effect known as the 'negative calorie illusion', when placed next to an 'unhealthy' food item. There was an experiment that involved a picture of a standard cheeseburger and asked participants to estimate how many calories were contained in the burger. In a second part of the experiment, a picture of the exact same cheeseburger but now with the addition of three sticks of celery on the side was used, and participants were once again asked to estimate how many calories were contained in the burger. What happened was the three sticks of celery actually conveyed a 'negative calorie illusion' on the burger, with the participants in the second part of the experiment estimating that the burger had a lower caloric content then those in the first part of the experiment who were simply looking at the burger. The celery sticks had become an 'incidental virtuous food' and, in the minds of the participants, had subtracted calories away from the burger.[18]

When I first read that paper, I was slightly incredulous that it would work. As it turns out, the explanation for the phenomenon was overly simplistic, and aspects of it could not be replicated.[19] However, just have a wander around your favourite supermarket or grocery store, and look at the depictions of food on packaging, the so-called 'serving suggestions'. Breakfast cereal for instance, is always pictured in a bowl with strawberries. Who has strawberries with their cornflakes? No one! Or you might have a packet of instant ramen noodles (VERY calorically available), depicting a very delicious looking bowl of noodles with carrots and coriander. Other examples might have steak pictured with parsley, or scrambled eggs with chopped chives. These are all being used as 'incidental virtuous foods', in order to convey a negative calorie illusion. There are studies, at the moment, being done to try and pick apart the mechanism for this, and trying to empirically test if we do end up buying and eating more calories as a result of the illusion. These are studies currently being undertaken by academics. Yet the negative calorie illusion is already in use on food packaging and advertising all around the world. Would food manufacturers have really deployed this approach so widely if they had not already done the experiments themselves? Hey, I'm just asking the question all of you were thinking.

THE DESSERT STOMACH

Given the importance that eating enough has in keeping us alive, our brain has evolved strategies to make sure that it also feels 'good' or rewarding to eat; the *'ooooooo'* factor. This is easily illustrated by the all too familiar 'dessert stomach', when you are out for a meal. We have all been there. It is almost certain that by the end of the main course you would have fulfilled your metabolic needs for the day; these are the number of calories you have expended that day, and therefore needed to recoup. Yet when the dessert menu arrives, you order the chocolate cake, tarte tatin or crème brûlée.

The interesting question to ask, however, is why is it specific to desserts? If at the end of the main course, the waiter came up and said, 'More potatoes?' or 'More steak?' or 'More rice?' you would say 'No thanks, if I ate any more I would puke!' (or words to that effect . . . Mr Creosote, anyone?)

Yet, while feeling exactly the same, you would order and then eat the chocolate cake.

To answer this question, we have to look to evolution once again. Flashback to 50,000 years ago on the Serengeti, and you are dragging an antelope back to the village. Let us just say it has cost you, metabolically speaking, 2,000 calories to stalk, chase and bring down the antelope. When you get back to the village, you would clearly have to consume at least 2,000 calories to recoup your expenditure. But there is no guarantee that you would successfully get an antelope the next time out, so if you ONLY ate to your metabolic need, you wouldn't survive very long. That is when the hedonic part of the brain, which governs the feeling of reward (the *'ooooooooo'* factor) kicks in, driving you to eat more. But how do you get past the mechanical difficulty of a stomach packed full with 2,000 calories of venison? Your brain becomes more picky, it begins to crave foods that are more calorically dense and more calorically available, which are going to be foods high in free sugars and fat. What foods are high in free sugars and fat? Desserts.

Your dessert stomach is an evolutionary holdover from your days in the Serengeti, to make sure that even when full, you were still craving the right types of foods to ensure you were able to maximise your caloric intake at every meal, because there was never a guarantee of when the next meal would arrive. It kept us alive in regular feast–famine cycles, but has become toxic for many of us in the feast–feast environment of today.

By the way, the 'dessert stomach' isn't just some weird human phenomenon. Sure, clearly a lion is not going to be topping off their freshly killed antelope luncheon with a crème brûlée and a chilled muscat. But let's take grizzly bears during the salmon runs in the Pacific Northwest of America as an example. The grizzlies hit the salmon runs, which take place in the autumn, with the intention of storing as much fat as possible for the coming winter hibernation. When they first start, the bears eat pretty much the whole salmon. However, as they get more and more full, and store more and more fat, they switch to just eating the skin of the salmon and the thin layer of fat that lies underneath. They begin to change the caloric density of what they are eating to maximise storage of energy. So while it is not 'dessert', it is the same phenomenon that accounts for the dessert stomach in humans.

ARE ALL CALORIES EQUAL?

So are all calories equal? From a physics perspective, as a unit of energy, yes.

But as I've hopefully convinced you in this chapter, we don't eat pure units of energy. What we eat is food, and we then have to figure out a way of extracting the calories out of the food as efficiently as possible. This begins with how we prepare or cook the food, and then how our digestive systems handle the various macronutrients. Then we have to figure out what proportion of the energy to use immediately and what proportion to store. Where and how much of the excess energy we can store then has relevance to our health and well-being. On top of that, how hungry or full we feel as we are eating then changes the caloric density of the particular food we are craving at the time.

To paraphrase a great author, yes, all calories are equal, but some are more equal than others.

PART 2

Palaeolithic dreams

Flintstones. Meet the Flintstones.
They're the modern stone-age family.

Theme tune to *The Flintstones* – 1960s

CHAPTER 4

Should we eat like the Flintstones?

I love BBQs. I love geeking out over the gear, I love the smell of lighter fluid over charcoal, I love the food, I love the cold beer, I love dining *al fresco* . . . despite the fact I left California 25 years ago and now live in a small village 10 miles outside of decidedly less sunny Cambridge. It's also never too early or late in the year to grill! I can be found outside, wrapped up in a fleece, scarf, woollen mittens and a beanie, breath visible in the crisp late February air, lighting charcoal for ribeye steaks.

'It's nearly spring!' I always tell my wife, while she looks at me through the patio door, shaking her head.

Every year, on the first weekend in May (which is always a three-day weekend here in the UK), my wife and I hold a BBQ in our backyard for friends and colleagues, as well as their partners and children. As it so happens, since I popped into the world on 1 May, the whole affair also doubles as my annual birthday celebration. I pride myself in preparing, marinating and cooking all of the food for the seventy or so hungry mouths that typically show up. A couple of years back, as I was manhandling a stack of baby-back ribs on to the grill, one of my friends, while clutching a beer in one hand (drinks always flow freely at the Yeo Birthday BBQ) and a teriyaki chicken wing in the other, shouted out:

'Hey, it's like watching Fred Flintstone with his Brontosaurus ribs! Are you trying to get all of us onto the Paleo diet?'

I guess if a Paleo diet means grilled meats in a sweet marinade, potato salad, sourdough bread and cold beer, then yes! However, aside from the presence of grilled meat (even then it has to be specific cuts of meat), everything else I've suggested is actually the antithesis of 'Paleo'. The sugar found in most BBQ marinades and sauces, potatoes, wheat flour in the bread as well as alcohol are all to be avoided like the plague if you are a Paleo enthusiast.

There are many people who assert we should be eating a Paleo diet. Are they right?

A 'STONE-AGE' DIET

The term 'Paleo' is a contraction of Palaeolithic, which is a prehistoric period going from about 2.6 million years ago (wayyyyy before *Homo sapiens* were walking about and around the time of *Homo habilis* or 'handy man') to 10,000 BC, and was characterised by, amongst other things, the development of stone tools. Hence, it is often colloquially referred to as 'The Stone Age'. The end of the Palaeolithic era also corresponded with the end of the Pleistocene, or 'Ice Age', and the beginning of the agricultural revolution. While it was first proposed by Dr Walter L. Voegtlin in his 1975 book *The Stone Age Diet*,[1] the Paleo diet as it exists today entered the popular consciousness in 2002, thanks to Dr Loren Cordain's bestselling book *The Paleo Diet: Lose Weight and Get Healthy by Eating the Foods You Were Designed to Eat*.[2] The diet was so named because it was designed to mimic the diet of indigenous populations prior to the agricultural revolution. The basic premise for the whole Paleo movement was that for the vast majority of human existence, since *Homo sapiens* emerged 200,000–300,000 years ago, we subsisted as hunter-gatherers. Then the dawn of the agricultural revolution some 12,000 years ago brought about huge changes to our diet. Since diet-related illnesses are responsible for much of the chronic and non-communicable disease burden today, and no evidence of such conditions can be seen in the Palaeolithic skeletal record, the blame for our contemporary woes must lie with the post-agricultural diet. Hence, according to Cordain, the solution to a skinnier and less-is-healthier human species must surely be to shift back to a pre-agricultural, so-called 'ancestral', subsistence.

Cordain developed this 'ancestral' diet, which he coined 'The Paleo Diet', using evidence from the fossil records, diets consumed by contemporary hunter-gatherer, chimpanzee diets and nutrients in wild animals and plants. He argued that in contrast to the modern western diet, Palaeolithic people hardly ever ate cereal grains, did not drink or eat dairy products, did not salt their food and the only sugar they ate was honey and only rarely and in small amounts. Instead, Palaeolithic diets were dominated by wild, lean animal meat and foods low in carbohydrate content; what little carbohydrates that were consumed came from non-starchy wild fruits and vegetables; and the staple fats in Palaeolithic diets were monounsaturated, polyunsaturated and omega 3 fats, found largely in plants and fish.

A central tenet to Cordain's philosophy is that the foods eaten (and not eaten) by ancient hunter-gatherer populations ensured optimal health due to the food's compatibility with the human genome. Cordain argues that those who adopt the Paleo diet will feel good 'because it is the only diet that is consistent with [the human] genetic makeup'.[3] Based on DNA evidence, he claims that basic human physiology has not changed significantly in 40,000 years, making our genes well adapted to a hunter-gatherer and NOT an agricultural lifestyle. Cordain claims that by switching to (or is it back to?) a Paleo lifestyle, we have the potential to control and even prevent diseases such as type 2 diabetes and insulin resistance, multiple sclerosis, rheumatoid arthritis, coeliac disease, cancer, heart disease, inflammation, osteoporosis and anaemia. In fact, he goes further, repeatedly stating that there are 'very few chronic illnesses or diseases that do not respond favourably to our ancestral diet, the diet to which our species is genetically adapted'.[4] These are very bold claims indeed.

Aficionados, of which there are many, can and will quote chapter and verse about the intricacies of the Paleo lifestyle or diet.[5] However, these can, by and large, be condensed into two basic sets of ground rules that you need to follow:

a) what you SHOULD eat is lean meat and seafood, as well as fruit and non-starchy vegetables, which can be consumed without limitation;

b) what you SHOULD NOT eat are cereals, legumes, dairy products and processed foods.

Just a note. We all know what grains from grasses are; so wheat, rice, oats and barley, etc. However, just in case, like me, you feel the need to look up what a legume is, its fruit is sometimes also referred to as a 'pod', and develops from a simple carpel, usually opening along a seam on two sides. The grain seed inside these 'pods' are known as pulses, which includes all beans, and also encompasses lentils, peas, peanuts and tamarind.

AGRICULTURE: EVOLUTION OR DEVOLUTION?

It is almost impossible to overstate the role that the agricultural revolution played in the development of human civilisation, for better and for worse, as it exists today. Because hunter-gatherers foraged all of their food, relying on what was in relatively close proximity, they had to follow the food and were therefore largely nomadic, or certainly at least semi-nomadic. Agriculture meant far higher food yields at predictable intervals, which allowed for the accumulation of stored food and a movement away from a nomadic lifestyle as well as the ability to support higher population densities. Hunter-gatherers, because of the inherent unpredictability of their food supplies, would have needed to devote most of their waking time to foraging and hunting. A predictable food supply afforded by farming, however, allowed for the emergence of non-food specialists in society. This was crucial because, all of a sudden, humans had the luxury of using their big brain for something else other than devising hunting strategy, finding out where the edible roots and berries were, and trying not to get killed or eaten. It turns out, in fact, that this availability of spare neuronal processing capacity, more than any other factor, was the central requirement for the subsequent development of all complex thoughts, concepts and technology. It is pretty difficult to contemplate quantum mechanics or cosmology, for instance, if you don't know where your next meal is coming from; so do remember to pass on a silent thanks to your proto-farmer ancestor as you order a pizza from your couch, using your smartphone. Another consequence of people beginning to specialise and do different things was that it drove the stratification of society. This stratification inevitably led to an 'upper' class (the people who owned the land and ate the food) wanting to control a 'lower' class (the people who were paid, or made, to produce the food). As villages grew into towns and towns into cities, centralised states and religions emerged, across the globe, as effective and efficient methods to control large populations. The next natural step was then the raising of armies of professional soldiers to defend and propagate state and religion, and here we are today. Hurrah for progress.

How we got into the mess we are in today, however, is not the main topic of discussion here. Let's rewind ourselves back 12,000 years to the dawn of agriculture. The truth of the matter is that Cordain was right that the transition from hunter-gatherer to farmer was not smooth at all. We know this from the archaeological evidence. Agriculture emerged independently in at least three different geographical locations. Emmer and Einkorn wheat was domesticated in the fertile crescent (a crescent-shaped area of fertile land along the River Nile in Egypt and the Tigris and Euphrates rivers in Mesopotamia) 10,000–12,500 years ago;[6] rice or *Oryza sativa* was thought to be domesticated in the Yangtze River Valley (although the exact location remains hotly debated, with the Pearl River Valley also staking a claim) in China some 9,000 years ago;[7] and maize or corn or *Zea mays* was domesticated from Mexican wild grass in the south of the country, also around 9,000–10,000 years ago.[8] According to a study of human remains from all of these areas, the height of the average person declined by 3 inches or more during the millennia in which the cultivation of each of these crops intensified.[9]

Our early farming ancestors were not just shorter than hunter-gatherers, indicating malnutrition and problems with growth, their skeletons also revealed a whole host of other illnesses. They had terrible dental problems, for example, with the incidence of cavities jumping nearly six-fold as people started relying on grain. One of the main issues with agriculture was that it resulted in a stunning reduction in the diversity of foods that we as humans ate, and consequently forced a huge shift in the sources from which we obtain our calories. Our continued reliance on the starch-rich seeds from five different grasses as our main source of calories is a perfect case in point. A second issue is the appearance of entirely new sources of food that were only possible after the establishment of agriculture. Consumption of milk and dairy products, for example, would only have made sense once herd animals had been domesticated. And likewise, the fermentation of fruit and grain to produce alcoholic beverages would only have been possible if there was an excess of such foods. The early farmers clearly had major problems adapting to this shift in diet.

The rapid increase in population density enabled by farming also resulted in a huge increase in infectious disease.[10] Diseases like measles, which, in the past, would have occurred in isolated nomadic pockets and then fizzled out, now had whole villages and towns of warm bodies, coughing, sneezing and spewing all manner of fluids, to aid their propagation. In addition, domestication brought large numbers of animals into close proximity with humans for the first time, allowing so-called 'zoonotic' diseases to jump between animals and humans. (These include common diseases such as the flu and chicken pox, to ones that cause more alarm like HIV and Ebola.)

Yet the advantages of agriculture to the growth and proliferation of our species were just too great, and so humans, flexible as we are, eventually adapted. The question is, however, were these adaptations at a detriment to our health? And if so, is the Paleo diet therefore the panacea to our modern-day problems of obesity and other metabolic diseases?

In order to answer these questions, let's take some of the major claims made by Cordain and other Paleo enthusiasts, and explore them in a little more detail.

1. OUR PALAEOLITHIC ANCESTORS ATE 'THE PALEO DIET'

The headline claim of the Paleo movement is that it has managed to replicate, or at the very least work out a reasonable facsimile of, what Palaeolithic people would have eaten. How true is this likely to be?

First, although Cordain is adamant about the specific foods and ratios in which they were consumed by hunter-gatherers, there are many that disagree with him. Randolph Nesse, the so-called godfather of evolutionary medicine, professor and director of the

Centre for Evolution & Medicine at Arizona State University, and author of many influential papers exploring the links between evolution and disease, finds the Paleo Diet simplistic and flawed. In an interview with NPR's (National Public Radio) Eliza Barclay, Nesse said:

'There's this tendency to want to find the normal human diet, but every single diet you pick has an advantage of some sort. Humans have lived in all kinds of places and we have adapted to all kinds of diets.'[11]

In a letter to the editor addressing a study published by Cordain and his colleagues in *The American Journal of Clinical* Nutrition,[12] Katherine Milton from the University of California at Berkeley stated that, 'hunter-gatherer societies, both recent and ancestral, displayed a wide variety of plant–animal subsistence ratios, illustrating the adaptability of human metabolism to a broad range of energy substrates. Because all hunter-gatherer societies are largely free of chronic disease, there seems little justification for advocating the therapeutic merits of one type of hunter-gatherer diet over another.'[13]

Peter Ungar and his colleagues, in the *Annual Review of Anthropology* reasoned that early *Homo* species would have had an adaptable and flexible diet, enabling them to survive in changing and unpredictable environments.[14] This does not necessarily mean that the foods they ate were varying all the time, but that they had the capacity to gain sustenance from many sources. This is really the bottom line, that there was no single Palaeolithic diet, because there was no singular Palaeolithic people. Rather, most experts agree that hunter-gatherers ate what was available to them at the time, depending on their environment.

Second, while the Paleo lifestyle condemns (and this really is not too strong a word here) foods that are a product of agriculture, the number of available foods that are NOT the product of agriculture, in one way or another, is actually extremely rare.

The vast majority of foods we eat today have been subject to years of genetic selection. Just to be crystal clear, I don't mean that everything we eat has been modified using modern genetic-engineering techniques. These are so-called GM foods, which I don't, in principle, have a problem with, while acknowledging we need to take care and attention with such powerful technology (I will discuss this in further detail in the final chapter). Rather, I refer to the fact that humans have been breeding plants and animals for the past 12,000 years. Farming has allowed humans to gradually alter plants to be more nutritionally dense, less toxic, larger and resistant to pests. Some examples include the domestication of the tomato, which has been bred to no longer contain toxins found in nightshade vegetables (whew!), or the evolution of apricots and almonds, which were bred from the same precursor; one to rear a larger fruit, the other an edible seed (I know! This was news to me too!). Apples are the products of hundreds of generations of careful breeding that started with a tree native to Central Asia, *Malus sieversii*. The author Michael Pollan once described those original fruit as tasting like 'a tart potato'.[15] Even avocados, the seemingly 'go-to' food for the clean-eating Instagram generation, have similarly been transformed from the original fruit, which consisted of just a thin layer of flesh surrounding a giant seed, to the delicious and creamy guacamole precursor of today. Almost every vegetable and fruit that we consume today would have undergone similar selection, to amplify their desirable traits and minimise the undesirable.

Similarly, the meat section in our supermarkets would be entirely foreign to our Palaeolithic ancestors. The busty, short-legged chickens of today are a far cry from the stringy, long-legged jungle fowl from which they were originally bred. All of our beef and dairy cattle are descended from the now-extinct aurochs, which were much larger and fiercer animals. On a recent trip to the University of Otago, in Dunedin, New Zealand, I happened upon a life-sized model of a Moa, a now extinct indigenous flightless bird that reached 3.6 metres in height. The size of the model was jaw-dropping. New Zealand was originally settled by humans around 1280 AD. Until that time, the Moa had no known natural predators, and so had no reason to fear these strange small hairless creatures that jumped off wooden boats and on to the beaches. From the point of view of those original Polynesian settlers, these birds were like a walking picnic, larder and restaurant wrapped up in one. Because they were not afraid of humans, the Polynesians simply walked up to them, poked them with a sharp stick, and boy, were they tasty. So much so that by 1400 AD, some 120 years after the arrival of the original human settlers, the Moas had been completely wiped out. 120 years, barely three generations, was all it took. Like the mammoths, mastodons and aurochs before, our ancestors hunted them to extinction. As Marlene Zuk writes in her book *Paleofantasy*, 'The reality is that we are not eating what our ancestors ate, perhaps because we do not want to, but also because we can't.'[16]

2. HUMANS EVOLVED TO EAT MEAT

The 'Paleo lifestyle' prescribes a diet high in protein, mostly from lean 'wild' or game meat and seafood, so the pork 'brontosaurus' ribs at my May BBQ, which I will attest do not fall into the 'lean' category, might not exactly fit the bill. However, there is a clear belief amongst the Paleo community that humans were evolved to eat primarily meat. Christina Warinner, an archeological scientist, gave an informative and revealing TED talk in 2013,[17] where she asserted that humans have few adaptations, genetic or otherwise, for meat consumption, but are actually physically adapted for plant consumption. These adaptations include a long digestive tract for plant digestion and the inability to produce vitamin C (not an asset, but evidence for the importance of plant consumption nonetheless). Carnivores, on the contrary, have shorter digestive tracts and have no need to ingest vitamin C, as they are able to create their own. They also have specific metabolic adaptations to an all-meat diet, such as the inability to synthesise vitamin A. In addition, Milton remarked that it was true that some Palaeolithic societies would have consumed large quantities of animal protein by today's standards, but 'this does not imply that such a dietary pattern is the most appropriate for human metabolism or that it should be emulated today.'[18] She stated that human gut proportions, as mentioned by Warinner, indicated a varied diet with digestion occurring primarily in the small intestine. Meat is, by far, more calorically dense than many vegetables. When this was coupled with the ability to control fire and the development of cooking techniques, the caloric availability of meat was incredibly valuable to Palaeolithic humans. However, chasing down meat was high-risk and hard-work, whereas the gathering of fruit, vegetables and roots was a more guaranteed source of food. Humans didn't evolve to eat ONLY meat, we evolved to eat whatever was available, including meat. Thus the fact that humans were omnivorous, with the ability to subsist on a hugely varied diet, was a key factor in our success as a species.

3. PROCESSED FOODS ARE BAD FOR YOU

On the face of it, saying that processed foods are bad for us does not seem to be a controversial statement. It certainly brings to mind the vast midsections of our favourite supermarkets that are set aside for processed confectioneries to suit all tastes. Whole aisles of breakfast cereals, chocolates and other candy, ready to leap on us and make us fatter. There are foods available whose shelf lives laugh in the face of going stale, almost defying biological decay and decomposition. A common urban myth claims that the infamous American 'cake' (a very loosely used term here I would argue), the Twinkie, has an infinite shelf life, due to all of the chemicals used in their production. In homage to this legend, the Pixar film *WALL-E*, which is set in part on a 'post-apocalyptic' Earth, has a scene where a cockroach is shown eating its way through the cream-filled centre of a Twinkie, both of which have survived the apocalypse, emerging out the other side not having been struck down by food poisoning. The myth is just that of course – a myth – but Twinkies certainly stay 'edible' (another word used here with great artistic license) for an unnaturally long time, particularly as they are filled with 'cream' (or at least some kind of cream analogue . . . what in heavens is in Twinkie cream?). In a less apocryphal tale, I was teaching at the Cuernavaca campus of the Universidad Nacional Autónoma de Mexico (UNAM) a few years ago, and was introduced, for the first time, to actual *bona fide* corn tortillas. They were delicious and made fresh to order, wherever they were served; be it as a street-food, or as fine dining in a Michelin-starred establishment. They have next to no shelf life at all, and are discarded if not eaten within the hour. 'Corn tortillas' are also available at my local supermarket, where I buy them to accompany my famous (at least within my household) chicken and steak fajitas. While these look like tortillas, they are a different beast entirely, and when kept sealed in the packaging they are sold in, have a shelf life of more than a year. If you think I jest, go check it out for yourselves! When I told my Mexican hosts about these 'tortillas', they stared at me in disbelief and said: 'Then they are not tortillas!'

The term 'processed', however, is a broad church. Cooking, for example, is by definition a 'process' which sterilises food and increases caloric availability. Is cooking bad for you? Clearly not. Heat treatment is also used as a process of preservation. Pasteurisation, for instance, heats milk (and other liquids) up to

60°C–72°C (140°F–161°F) for a few seconds, killing off the majority of microbes without impairing flavour, and extending the shelf life of milk from a couple of days to two weeks or more. The US Center for Disease Control (CDC) says that improperly handled raw milk is responsible for nearly three times more hospitalisations than any other food-borne disease source, making it one of the world's most dangerous food products. Hurrah for pasteurisation!

As well as this, putting heat-treated food into a heat-sterilised container and then sealing it, as happens during the canning process or when one is making jam, extends its shelf life indefinitely, often without the use of any preservatives, aside from sugar or vinegar.

The processing of food, prior to the advent of refrigeration, was almost always used as a form of preservation. Curing is probably the oldest such example, and has been the dominant method of meat preservation for thousands of years. Meat or fish were most commonly cured by the addition of salt or sugar or a combination of both, with the aim of drawing moisture out of the food by the process of osmosis. The resulting decrease in moisture content and increase of salt and/or sugar concentration within the meat makes it an inhospitable environment for the bacteria that causes food to spoil. Smoking is often performed in conjunction with the addition of salt, helping to seal the outer layer of the food being cured, and making it more difficult for bacteria to enter. Thus emerged bacon, ham, salami and a whole menagerie of smoked fish, including salmon, haddock and mackerel. Dehydration, by simply drying food out in the sun (beef jerky, anyone?), is another of the earliest forms of food preservation and works because bacterial growth requires water.

Fermentation is a food preservation method using microorganisms. Examples include any process that produces alcoholic beverages or acidic dairy products, for instance, and involves either yeast or specific types of bacteria converting sugars into lactic acid or alcohol. The earliest documented use of fermentation dates back to nearly 7000 BC in Jiahu, China, where the first evidence of an alcoholic drink made from the fermentation of fruit was discovered.[19] Yogurt, which is produced by the bacterial fermentation of milk, converting lactose to lactic acid, was thought to have been invented in Mesopotamia around 5000 BC.[20] Fermentation has also been used as a method of preserving vegetables in many cultures, with examples of fermented cabbage that include sauerkraut in Europe and kimchi in Korea.

Then there are processes that involve separation, such as the milling of rice or wheat, which is where it has its husk, bran and germ removed. The act of polishing after milling is what gives rice its characteristic white colour, its taste and texture. Crucially this refining of rice extended the storage life of the dried grain, which would presumably have been the primary reason why it was developed. Unfortunately, an unintended consequence of this refining is that much of the nutritional content of rice, which is actually contained within the husk, is removed. In fact, a diet based on unenriched white rice increases vulnerability to the neurological disease 'beriberi', due to a deficiency of vitamin B1 or thiamine. Today, in an effort to replace some of the nutrients stripped from it during its processing, white rice is required by law, at least in the United States, to be enriched with vitamins B1, B3 and iron.

Another ancient process is the practice by indigenous peoples in the Americas of soaking corn in an alkaline solution, typically lime (not the fruit but the mineral), prior to cooking. Before the arrival of Europeans, corn would have been the primary grain in the Americas. It still is the primary grain in many parts of Central and South America today. The problem with corn is that while it is particularly rich in the micronutrient niacin, otherwise known as vitamin B3, the niacin is chemically unavailable to the human digestive system, and passes right through us. So if the grain you ate was primarily corn, you could end up with niacin deficiency, resulting in a disease called pellagra, which is characterised by diarrhoea, dementia, rash on the hands and feet, and if left untreated, is lethal. Soaking the corn in alkaline solution liberated the niacin, making it available to us during digestion. How the indigenous Americans worked it out is a mystery, but seeing as corn was domesticated some 10,000 years ago, work it out through trial and error they did, and pellagra was never a problem for them. After the arrival of Europeans, corn was very quickly adopted by the colonial Europeans and also exported to Europe. None of the Europeans or white Americans, however, picked up on the alkali treatment of corn prior to cooking, or if they did, they certainly didn't grasp the significance of that process. For most non-native Americans, the unavailability of niacin from corn was not a problem, because niacin was available from other sources of food, including meat and other grains. However, corn was cheap and easy to grow, so ended up being a primary staple to those in poverty, causing a sharp increase in incidence of pellagra amongst the poor. It wasn't until the mid-1930s and early 1940s that pellagra was recognised as a disease resulting from niacin deficiency and eradicated by the fortification of grains and flour. Imagine that: corn had been around for nearly 10,000 years, and it took non-native Americans and Europeans until the early twentieth century to learn how to process it properly for food.[21]

So while the term 'processed food', as used today, is associated with a whole host of negative connotations, the devil truly is in the detail. Clearly, the modern industrial processes giving rise to Twinkies and mutant corn tortillas have extended the shelf life of food, sometimes indefinitely, making transport and storage far easier, and, importantly, driving down their cost. These are critical characteristics of contemporary food that allow the planet to sustain its seven billion human inhabitants and rising. However, while calories today in most developed economies are plentiful and cheap, highly industrially processed foods are typically stripped of much of their nutrients and fibre, contain higher levels of sugar, fat and/or salt in order to improve flavour, and are as a consequence far more calorically available. However, food preservation and separation processes were critical to our ability as a species to survive and to thrive, ensuring that we had a predictable source of calories through seasonal changes in the availability of fresh food, and buffering against environmental crises such as drought. So depending on how one defines it, we can't – and shouldn't – avoid all processed foods.

4. OUR GENES ARE NOT ADAPTED TO THE POST-AGRICULTURAL DIET

The claim that our genes are not adapted to the post-agricultural diet is one that is possibly used the most by Paleo enthusiasts. It is also the most nuanced, particularly as a key argument which I make is that our food environment has changed too quickly for our genes to adapt, leading to the current obesity epidemic. Before I am accused of providing 'alternative facts', let me explain. The environmental changes that I spoke about in the beginning of this book, which include changes in food availability, type of food, as well as changes to our lifestyle, have occurred in the past thirty years. This is far too short a time for us to have genetically adapted. In contrast, humans have been exposed to agriculture now for thousands of years and, given the selection pressure the environment has provided, have had ample time and opportunity to genetically adapt to it. Two informative examples have been our adaptation to handle an increased volume of starch and our ability to drink and metabolise alcohol.

The other aspect to consider is whether it's true that our Palaeolithic ancestors did not eat grains. Today, the starchy rich seeds of five grasses (wheat, rice, oats, corn and barley) provide 50 per cent of the calories consumed by all humans. This is certainly very different from what our Palaeolithic hunter-gatherer ancestors would have faced. However, Anna Revedin, an archaeologist at the Italian Institute of Prehistory, found that grinding stones were used to process wild cereals and ground seeds as far back as 30,000 years ago.[22] By examining starch grains recovered from the grinding stones found at three Palaeolithic sites across Europe, they concluded that early Palaeolithic populations made flour, allowing them to consume the starch-rich portions of otherwise inedible plants and providing a more dependable food source. They also suggest that their findings indicate the use of this type of food processing would have been relatively common practice throughout European Palaeolithic hunter-gatherers. What is now clear is that the technology to convert inedible grain into energy-rich flour predated the agricultural 'big bang' by nearly 20,000 years. While Palaeolithic people were certainly not exposed to the same volume of the five starch-rich grasses that we see today, it is patently untrue that they did not consume grains as food.

The problem is with the amount of grains, and hence starch, that was suddenly available. Our foraging ancestors in the Pleistocene may have occasionally happened upon a field of early wheat or rice, but their caloric base would have come from a huge variety of foods, nuts, berries and game.

In humans, our ability to digest starch begins with amylase in saliva, which helps break down starch during chewing, and continues its action as it travels down to the stomach, and through to the small intestine, where other amylases released from the pancreas and other organs take over. Although we typically carry two copies of any given gene, one from each parent, humans actually have a variable number of the saliva amylase gene AMY1, ranging from 2 to more than 30 copies. The more copies of AMY1, the better our ability to digest starch. This improvement in ability is subtle but measurable. Genetic studies on existing hunter-gatherer peoples today, such as the Yanomami people of Venezuela, who continue to subsist on a high protein and low starch diet, reveal they have fewer copies of AMY1; while other primates, who are primarily fruit eaters, only ever have 2 copies of AMY1.[23]

Humans have always eaten starch, we just were not able to fully digest it and unlock all of the available calories. This was not a problem when starch was not our overwhelming source of calories (such as for the Yanomami), which it is, of course, today. What this genetic adaptation has done is to improve our efficiency to metabolise starch, allowing us to extract more calories from every gram of starch. Or to look at it another way, we could eat less food and get the same number of calories. Even in the relatively plentiful environment post the agricultural 'big bang', at least in comparison to the scrabbling existence of hunting and gathering, most humans still didn't have a surfeit of available food. An increased efficiency to digest starch provided a huge selective advantage over those without the genetic adaptation, and was therefore incorporated into the gene-pool, such that almost all humans today carry multiple copies of AMY1.

Our shift to a starch-rich diet had one other unintended consequence that ended up significantly influencing human culture; it was a major driving factor in the domestication of dogs. Dogs were domesticated from wolves 10,000–20,000 years ago, possibly multiple times independently. Dogs don't have salivary amylase, but have an amylase that is produced by the pancreas called AMY2B. Similar to AMY1 in humans, dogs have a variable number of AMY2B genes, with more copies indicating a better ability to digest starch.[24] Wolves, however, only appear to have 2 copies of AMY2B. Together with a less vicious disposition, the enhanced ability of the ancestors of modern dogs to digest starch led to them being able to subsist off human starch-rich food waste, which would have been a valuable source of energy, and they were therefore less likely to eat their human companions (that would not have worked out). People often assume that dogs are 'obligate' carnivores, a fact which is true for wolves and indeed cats. However, a peek at the ingredient list of any brand of packaged dog-food will reveal a surprisingly high starch content, a diet which our dogs are genetically adapted to!

Alcohol

On a lovely October's day at the turn of the millennium, I married the love of my life (Jane) here in Cambridge. We were married at the Catholic Church in the centre of town, and then booked out a large local Chinese restaurant for our wedding banquet. My wife is English and largely of Northern European extract, with about an eighth Irish thrown into the mix. As a result, the guests in attendance were about 40 per cent Chinese (groom's side), 50 per cent white Caucasian (bride's side) and 10 per cent of every shade and colour else (our academic colleagues from all corners of the world). In addition to the food on offer, which catered to all the dietary needs you might imagine, there was of course a typical selection of beer, wine and non-alcoholic drinks, and as it was a wedding reception in the UK after all, copious amounts of champagne were also on offer. Some guests, particularly from my wife's side of the family, enjoyed more than a few drinks (it was a wedding after all!), the volume of conversation and laughter growing louder as the afternoon merged into the evening. Others (primarily on my side of the family) drank little, if at all. Many of my family simply have an inability to metabolise alcohol, evident by the flushed cheeks on display after only a few sips of bubbles, and also a boisterous contribution to the conversation and laughter. So why are there differences in the way we metabolise alcohol, and how has its consumption, or lack thereof, become so culturally entrenched?

Alcohol is broken down in the body by a number of alcohol dehydrogenases (ADHs). The oldest forms of ADH4, found in primates some 50 million years ago, broke down small amounts of alcohol very slowly and inefficiently. About 10 million years ago, however, a single genetic mutation occurred that enabled a common ancestor of humans, chimpanzees and gorillas to develop a version of the ADH4 protein that was 40 times more efficient at metabolising alcohol.[25] This abrupt shift occurred at a time of rapid climate change, causing the forest ecosystem of East Africa, home of our primate ancestors, to be replaced by more widely dispersed forests and grasslands. While early primates had lived their lives mostly in trees, as the environment and food sources began to change, some of them made the transition to a more ground-based lifestyle.

Crucially, the new ability to digest alcohol helped our ground-dwelling primate ancestors eat rotting and fermenting fruit (which were alcoholic) that fell to the floor of the forest when other food was scarce. Such fallen fruit would have been unlikely to be the first choice of food, but it would have allowed them to survive. Other primates without this mutation were more likely to get sick or drunk off the fermented fruit, and be less effective at defending their territory or finding more food. Thus all primates that live primarily on the ground (including us) can handle a small amount of alcohol.

The embedding of alcohol into our culture, however, came with the emergence of agriculture. According to archaeological evidence, the first modern humans began turning fermented fruit and other foods into alcoholic concoctions at the beginning of the agricultural revolution. Critically, this then influenced the strategy of how certain populations solved the problem of safe drinking water. Alcohol, in the form of beer and wine, was used by those in the fertile crescent (today's Middle East) and northern Europe to ensure safe drinking water. Thus an enhanced ability to metabolise alcohol, the result of another single gene mutation, was a hugely powerful selective advantage. In fact, European children regularly drank weak beer up until the 17th century.

Whereas for other cultures, in particular many East Asian and other indigenous cultures, the strategy of boiling water (eventually enhanced in flavour by the addition of local leaves to produce 'tea') was used instead. That is not to say that ancient East Asians did not drink alcohol. The residue of the earliest known alcoholic beverage (a mixed fermented drink of rice, honey and fruit) was actually found on early pottery used in Jiahu,[26] a Neolithic village in China's Yellow River Valley dating to 7000–6600 BC, slightly predating that of barley beer and grape wine, which emerged in the Middle East. However, because East Asians had clean boiled water, they didn't HAVE to drink alcohol, unlike the Northern Europeans in particular. Thus emerged the variation in the ability of different populations today to handle the drinking of alcohol.

Now let's return to my wedding, where the reception has now metamorphosed into a full 'wave your hands in the air'-type party. From a sociological perspective and given the diversity of nation-alities in attendance, it is interesting to note that, earlier in the proceedings, many guests felt the need to accept a small (or not so small) glass of champagne to toast the bride and groom, whether or not they could drink any of it, because it is the culturally accept-able thing to do. This is hardly unique to my wedding. Economic globalisation has led to the emergence of a large middle class with expendable income in places like China and India, where both at home and abroad they are exposed to western culture. For better or worse, a part of this involves the adoption of western drinking culture as a status symbol; what could be more 'cultured' than a glass of champagne at a wedding in Cambridge?!

Now, alcohol is actually a toxin, which is why it is used to ster-ilise drinking water. Drinking alcohol in moderate amounts is not a problem for those who can metabolise it, thus removing it rapidly from the blood. The problem is, if one lacks the ability to remove alcohol from the blood, like many of my family and East Asian colleagues, then the alcohol remains circulating as a toxin, where even at moderately high concentrations, it can be as carcinogenic as smoking a pack of cigarettes. A small snifter of champagne at a chimeric English–Chinese wedding is not going to kill anyone. But it is best to be aware of what our bodies are designed to eat and drink.

The point is, if there is a strong enough selection pressure, then genetic adaptations, such as an increased efficiency of starch digestion or the ability to drink alcohol, can take place over a relatively short period of time.

A beer belly segue

One thing that many people don't take into consideration is the caloric content of alcoholic beverages; not an issue at all for folks like my dad, however a particular problem for those that can drink like fish. But surely it's only beer that contains lots of carbs and therefore lots of calories? Isn't that why all of those loud and sweaty men (I am channelling my wife here for a moment) who swill beer the world over have beer bellies? I mean, look at all of those skinny ladies drinking prosecco . . .

Here's the thing. When it comes to alcohol and weight gain, the term 'beer belly' is misleading. The majority of calories from drinking don't come from the carbs, they come from the alcohol. Pure alcohol, at seven calories per gram, contains almost the same amount of calories as fat (9 calories per gram), and is no more or less calorific whatever drink it happens to be in; whether it is beer, wine, gin or whisky. So, a 175ml glass of wine, with an alcohol content of 13 per cent, contains nearly 160 calories, while a whole bottle will be around 700 calories. A standard 330ml bottle of beer with 5 per cent alcohol contains 140 calories, while the equivalent in a UK pint will be over 240 calories. Compare this to 140 calories found in a can of Coca-Cola and 250 calories found in a Snickers or Mars bar. Very few people would consume six cans of cola in one sitting, whereas many would think nothing of drinking a six-pack of beer. In addition, there are many alcoholic drinks, mixers or alcopops, for instance, that are also high in sugar, jacking up the calorie content even further. And the denouement is that the more you drink, the more disinhibited you become, and the less you will care about what and how much you are consuming. An evening out could easily lead to 700–1,000 calories just in drinks, before you even consider any food you have eaten.

Any spare calories you don't use immediately will then be converted in to fat. Where you put your fat depends on your own personal biology. As we've discussed, on average, men are more likely to store theirs in visceral fat that sits around their belly (hence beer belly), while women will tend to store it underneath their skin as subcutaneous fat. So it's just less obvious in a woman ... although perhaps we could coin the term 'wine wobble', or maybe 'champagne chin'?

But I digress. The Paleo diet is a made-up construct because what we might have eaten in the Palaeolithic Age is always going to be a guess, and much of what we may have actually eaten probably doesn't exist in any recognisable form today anyway! And the arguments that we haven't genetically adapted to an agricultural diet simply make no sense, as I have just shown.

DO HIGH-PROTEIN, LOW-CARB DIETS WORK?

One of the key characteristics of the Paleo Diet is its prescribed high-protein and low-carbohydrate content. This however, is not unique to the Paleo world, and is shared by other diets including, amongst many others, the Dukan and Ketogenic diets, as well as the granddaddy of them all, the Atkins diet. I do realise that these are different diets with differing philosophies; and I am using the word 'philosophies' here with all the baggage that it comes with. Let's take a look at each of them in turn.

The Dukan diet has the ATTACK phase, which gives your weight loss a jump start; the CRUISE phase, which gets you down to your target weight; the CONSOLIDATION phase, which tries to prevent any immediate rebound; and the STABILISATION phase, which is the long-term strategy to keep the weight off.[27] It is clear that the Dukan diet has been heavily influenced by the Atkins diet, which is also divided into four phases: induction, ongoing weight loss, pre-maintenance and maintenance. In fact, at first glance, they might almost be the same diet.

This is what the Dukan diet claims to do. 'The Dukan Diet will redesign your eating habits and help you permanently stabilise your weight. The Dukan Diet is a high-protein, low-fat, low-carb diet – a healthy-eating plan based on proteins and vegetables, 100 foods in total. And what's best, it's EAT AS MUCH AS YOU LIKE.'[28] (There are those shouty capital letters again.) It really is quite a restrictive diet . . . only 100 foods you can eat, but without limit! The Atkins diet is nowhere near as prescriptive, really only limiting carbohydrate consumption, with protein and fat making up the rest of the diet. For both Dukan and Atkins, the main difference between the four phases is the protein to carb ratio of the diet; with phase 1 in both having the highest protein and lowest carb content.

The ketogenic diet is a high-fat, moderate-protein, very low-carbohydrate diet. It is so named because it forces the body to burn fat rather than carbohydrates, a process called ketosis, which produces ketone bodies as a by-product. In the clinical setting, it has been used for decades to treat particularly hard to control epilepsy in children. The exact mechanism is unknown, but by forcing the brain to use ketones as fuel rather than its favoured glucose, this seems to reduce the number of seizures that occur. It is, however, now beginning to gain traction as a weight-loss plan. While the ketogenic diet is sold as a high-fat, ultra-low-carb diet, the reality is that many people cannot manage the 75 per cent to 80 per cent fat that is recommended. It is an extreme level of fat that is quite unpalatable to many. Keto enthusiasts tend to come to the diet with an almost evangelical aim of avoiding carbs, and because the calories still need to come from somewhere, the diet actually ends up being quite high in protein; maybe as high as 20–25 per cent, as compared to the 15 per cent protein in today's typical western diet.

The reason that this common thread of high protein and low carb exists in many diets is because the approach does work, at least in the short term, for weight loss.

The main stumbling block is one that is universal to ALL diets; that is, the moment you come off the diet, the weight, almost invariably, goes back on. Why? Because your brain absolutely hates it when you lose even a few pounds, sensing weight loss as a danger signal, a warning that you need to maintain your energy stores. Your body fights back by reducing its energy expenditure and making you feel hungrier, in an effort to claw back the weight it has lost. So if you stop whatever diet you were on, and go back to how you were eating, your weight will soon climb back to where it was before you began the diet.

Then there are the myriad of side-effects to contend with on a ketogenic diet, depending on how extreme a protein to carb ratio you try to stick to. Heart palpitations, headaches, leg cramps, constipation and bad breath, for example, have all been reported as common side-effects. Taken to its most extreme, however, such as in untreated type 1 diabetes, where you don't have any insulin and thus your muscles and fat are unable to absorb any glucose, you would end up burning only fat, producing uncontrolled amounts of ketones, and ending up with diabetic ketoacidosis. Because ketone bodies are acidic, a large accumulation would dangerously lower the pH of the blood – thus the name ketoacidosis, which, if left unchecked, can be fatal. This, by the way, is my riposte to those who say we can live perfectly healthy lives without eating any carbohydrates and just use ketones from the breakdown of fat as fuel. Without at least some carbohydrates in our diet, we would die.

WHY DOES HIGH PROTEIN EQUAL WEIGHT LOSS?

But there is good evidence that a moderate increase in the protein to carb ratio works for weight loss. The question is why and how does it work? Most of the diets above, in their various website blurbs and glossy brochures, focus on the 'low-carb' element of the diet. There is an almost universal (although admittedly to varying degrees) condemnation of carbohydrates and agreement about their toxic nature; it is after all the food element that is being removed, or at least reduced drastically. How about the macronutrient that is being added, though? What about the role of increasing the amount of protein being eaten?

The first thing to consider is caloric availability, which we discussed in detail in Chapter 3. Protein takes the most energy and the longest time to digest, with nearly 30 per cent of the total calories eaten in protein required to digest it. Contrast this to carbohydrates, which only take 5–10 per cent of consumed calories to digest, depending on whether we're talking about complex starches, which would cost more, or simple sugars which would cost less. So calorie for calorie, it takes more energy to digest protein than carbohydrates.

But protein also makes you feel fuller than carbs or fat. Why? The answer to this question lies in our gut hormones and the biology of how they control our feeding behaviour.

GUT HORMONES

In order to effectively modulate our feeding behaviour, including how full or how hungry you might feel, your brain needs to know the answers to two critical questions. First, what is the state of your long-term energy stores? This is, broadly speaking, the amount of fat that you currently have on-board, which is how long you would last without food. Second, what is the state of your short-term energy stores? This would include what you are currently eating, what you have just eaten and how much is being consumed. As food travels from our mouths, down our oesophagus and through our gastrointestinal tract, hormones are released all along the way that reflect not only how many calories are in the meal, but also how much protein, fat and carbohydrates are present. The vast majority of hormones that are released by the stomach and gut, such as CCK, GLP-1 and PYY, make us feel full.[29] CCK or chole- cystokinin, for example, is released from the stomach and is very short acting, with its 'feel full' effect lasting less than 30 minutes; thus it is likely to play a role in signalling when you should stop eating. In contrast, PYY or peptide YY, which is secreted by the small and large intestine, has effects that last many hours, bridging the gap between meals, and therefore influencing how much you are likely to eat from one meal to the next. The one exception to the 'gut hormones make you eat less rule' is ghrelin, which is produced by the stomach, and makes us feel hungry.[30] In fact, ghrelin levels in the blood rise acutely just before a meal, triggering hunger and playing a role in when we choose to eat.[31] Your brain doesn't sense and respond to each of these hormones in isolation. Rather, it is a mix of these short and long acting signals (of which there are many more than just the four I've discussed here), as well as when and where they are released, that signals to the brain how much and what is being eaten.[32]

In recent years, our understanding of how these gut hormones modulate our feeding behaviour has been transformed by lessons learnt from gut bypass or bariatric surgery.[33]

WHY PROTEIN MAKES YOU FEEL FULL – LESSONS LEARNT FROM RE-PLUMBING THE GUT

Gut bypass or bariatric surgery is used as a weight-loss treatment for severe obesity. It is, in fact, the only current anti-obesity therapy that reliably keeps weight off in the long term. The observation of how obese people responded to gut-bypass surgery not only gave us a further appreciation of how the whole system was working, but also proved a plausible mechanism for how and why high-protein diets work in weight loss. There are a number of different types of bariatric surgery that exist, with the most commonly used being the Roux-en-Y gastric bypass or RYGB. By stapling off the upper section of the stomach, this surgery first reduces the size of the upper stomach to a small pouch of about 30 millilitres in volume; then the second stage sees this pouch being attached directly to a part of the small intestine lower down, bypassing about one metre of the upper small intestine, or duodenum. The surgery has, in effect, re-plumbed the gut. By making the stomach drastically smaller and bypassing a length of small intestine, RYGB was designed to limit the amount of food able to be consumed and to reduce the amount of fat and calories absorbed from the food that has been eaten. However, while RYGB was tremendously effective in reducing weight, HOW it worked turned out to be a big surprise.

Two key observations of patients pre- and post-RYGB have transformed our understanding of how the gut works. First, many of the obese people who underwent bariatric surgery also commonly suffered from type 2 diabetes. The doctors observed that after RYGB, the patients' diabetes improved dramatically; in many cases, patients could actually reduce or even stop their anti-diabetic medication. It was the speed at which this occurred that really surprised doctors, with improvements in diabetes happening less than twenty-four hours after the surgery, clearly before any notable weight loss could have occurred![34] Second, after the surgery, many patients reported a change in eating behaviour, once again beginning before any notable weight loss. Not only did they feel full faster, but their taste in food also changed.[35] Many found fatty foods less appealing, for instance.

So what was going on? Was the smaller stomach playing a major role? No, as it turns out. Because the stomach is very flexible, it begins to stretch quite rapidly, and before long, the same volume of food can fit into the stomach again. The major effects came from the bypass element of the surgery. Under normal circumstances, food leaves the stomach and enters the small intestine, where the bulk of digestion occurs. The lower down the intestine the food goes, the more digested the food gets, and all the while the intestine is secreting hormones to keep the brain informed of progress. The effect of the bypass is to introduce food that is in a different state, that has been slightly less digested, lower down the small intestine. This part of the gut that has been exposed to less digested food then responds by secreting a different mix of hormones. It is this different repertoire of hormones that resolves the diabetes, makes the patient feel more full and eat less.[36]

What does this have to do with how high-protein diets work? In a post-bariatric surgery gut, the bypass transfers less digested food further down the gut, which makes you feel fuller. Whereas in a higher-protein diet, because proteins are less calorically available and take longer to digest than fat and carbs, they end up travelling further down the gut, which, due to hormonal release, then makes you feel fuller. What happens when you feel full? You eat less. And what happens when you eat less? Well, it is the most effective way to lose weight.

LEVERAGING PROTEIN

The reason there is even a need for bariatric surgery and all of these diets is, of course, because of rapidly increasing rates of obesity and all of its associated diet-related illnesses. A major driver of this modern obesity crisis is our food environment, including, as I've discussed earlier in this chapter, the increased availability of industrially processed, calorically dense, yet nutrient-poor food. We are driven to eat these items because they are often rich in fat, sugar and/or salt, and are therefore highly palatable.

A different hypothesis has emerged in recent years that provides another possible reason why we might find these foods so palatable, and it revolves around the fact that these foods also tend to have a lower protein content. In 2005, writing in the journal *Obesity Reviews*, Australian scientists Stephen J. Simpson and David Raubenheimer from the University of Sydney proposed 'The Protein Leverage Hypothesis' as a possible driver of the obesity epidemic.[37] They argued that most emphasis on the dietary causes of obesity has been on our changing patterns of fat and carbohydrate consumption. Whereas the role of protein has been relatively ignored because it only comprises around 15 per cent of the western diet, and all available evidence points to protein intake remaining constant across multiple different populations, even in the face of rising obesity levels. So because protein intake hasn't changed, it couldn't be playing a role in the problem.

What if, however, a major driving force in what and how much we eat is to maintain a certain level of protein in our diet? In other words, even if protein only forms 15 per cent of our diet, what happens if we NEED it to be 15 per cent, because it is a critical level that we need to meet in order to survive?

Simpson and Raubenheimer conducted an initial small and short-term experiment to test their hypothesis.[38] They put ten volunteers into the same living space for six days. For the first two days, everyone was free to select all of their meals from a buffet comprising a wide range of foods with known macronutrient content. Everything they ate was weighed and the amount of protein, carbs and fat calculated. Then for the next two days (days three and four), one group of subjects (treatment 1) was restricted to foods that were high in protein and low in carbs, while the remaining volunteers (treatment group 2) were provided with only low protein and high carb items. Then on days five and six, everyone reverted to the free-choice buffet, as on days one and two. The results showed that when the subjects were restricted to a diet that contained either a higher (treatment 1) or lower (treatment 2) protein-to-carb ratio than they had self-selected during the first two days, they maintained their intake of protein at the expense of regulation of carbohydrate intake. In other words, treatment group 1 (high protein, low carb) ate fewer carbs rather than overeat protein, while treatment group 2 (low protein, high carb) overate carbs in order to get enough protein. Because the volunteers were subconsciously trying to achieve a specific level of protein rather than calories *per se* in their diet, the protein 'leveraged' the amount of carbs that they ended up eating; eating less of a high-protein, low-carb diet and more of a low-protein, high-carb diet. While this initial 2005 study was small and conducted over a short term, more evidence from human epidemiological studies, as well as studies in flies and mice, have emerged to support this hypothesis.

There are obvious and worrying implications for this 'protein leverage effect'. In the western world, obesity risk is inversely related to socio-economic class; to put it bluntly, it means that the poorer you are, the more likely you are to be obese or overweight. The reasons for this are varied, complex and, frankly, not entirely known. One explanation is that fast-food outlets and takeaways, which tend to sell cheap and highly processed food, are found at their highest densities in less affluent areas. Conversely, high protein foods such as fish and lean meat are relatively more expensive to those on lower incomes than to the more affluent. Many of you, as I was when I found out, will be surprised, shocked even, to know that 'food insecurity' is a serious problem here in the UK. In 2014, there were an estimated 8.4 million people in the UK, the world's sixth-largest economy, living in households reporting having insufficient food. That is the equivalent of the entire population of London or New York: just think about that for a minute. I am acutely aware that I am fortunate enough not to be 'food insecure', so I am not going to judge how someone on a limited budget chooses to feed his or her family. I am also not inferring causation; but the easy availability of cheap, highly processed food that tends to be lower in protein content is clearly part of a vicious cycle driving the obesity epidemic, and also exacerbating social inequality.

HOW SHOULD WE EAT?

But just so we are clear, it is not simply about protein, but about 'putting the balance back in diet'.[39] In 2015, Simpson and Raubenheimer, together with David Le Couteur, authored an essay in the journal *Cell*, in which they argue that 'the notion of dietary balance is fundamental to health yet is not captured by focusing on the intake of energy or single nutrients.'[40] This is a crucial point, given that we don't eat individual nutrients; rather, we eat food.

Let us take the fruit fly as an example. Fruit flies eat primarily protein and carbs, and hardly any fat at all. So they represent a simple model of testing out the physiological effect of altering the ratio of protein to carbs in their diet, and also what flies actually prefer to eat. If flies are made to eat specific diets, then the lower the protein to carb ratio of their diet (low protein, high carb), the longer the lifespan of a fly. Whereas a diet that maximised their reproductive success, but compromised on lifespan, had a far higher protein to carb ratio. What was really interesting was when allowed to choose what they preferred to eat, flies chose to mix a diet maximising reproductive output rather than lifespan. This makes an awful lot of sense, because the goal of all living beings, after all, is not to live as long as possible at all costs, but to live long enough to be reproductively successful, to be able to pass on their genes. Similar studies were performed on mice, but using protein to carb + fat ratios, and the same results emerged; the diet composition that best supported longevity was not the same as that which sustained maximal reproductive output. The bottom line is when given a choice, mice and flies choose diets that balance longevity with reproductive capability.[41] Put another way, mice and flies prefer to live fast and die young!

Clearly humans make dietary decisions for different reasons from mice and flies. However, in at least one respect, humans are not so different; we strive for balance. Fifteen per cent of protein in our diet is what we aim for, but the lower protein content in the industrial processed elements of our modern diet leverages us into eating too much, driving obesity, and shortening our lifespan. On the other end of the spectrum, multiple studies, including from the Nurses' Health Study, the Health Professionals' Follow-up Study, the Swedish Women's Health and Lifestyle cohort, and the Greek cohort of the European Prospective Investigation into Cancer and Nutrition, all consistently indicated that over a long term, low-carbohydrate and high-protein diets increased risk of diabetes, heart disease and mortality.[42]

So how should we eat? Well, with diets, as with most things in life, the most boring of messages continues to ring true; moderation is key.

CHAPTER 5

Good gluten, bad gluten and ugly gluten

The city of Cambridge is a beautiful place and has the advantage of being home to one of the oldest and most famous universities in the world. The University of Cambridge bore witness to and survived the Black Death, the Wars of the Roses, the Reformation and two world wars, celebrating its 800th birthday in 2009. It should, hopefully, be able to stand up against and navigate the 'post-truth' anti-intellectualism of today. The university is formed of thirty-one fiercely independent colleges and various academic departments dotted throughout the city. The older colleges are covered with immaculate lawns that have been rolled and mowed, and then rolled and mowed again for hundreds of years; not a sign of a weed will you see. The colleges are also filled with buildings made of actual stone (concrete is a dirty word in Cambridge), the walls crawling with ancient ivy; many of the old rooms are adorned with ornate panelling and furniture made with rich, dark wood, undoubtedly unsustainably sourced from years gone by. The oldest part of town is so ridiculously picturesque and quaint . . . Except, of course, that it is a place where people actually live, work and learn. Set further out, surrounding the old town in a ring, are the newer colleges. Wolfson College, where I was a graduate student and am now a fellow, is practically embryonic, having just turned fifty years young in 2015. It was at a black-tie affair to celebrate

Wolfson's fiftieth birth-year where this tale begins.

Formal dinners at a Cambridge college are, surprisingly, pretty accurately depicted in the *Harry Potter* books and movies; black-gowned scholars sitting at multiple rows of long wooden tables lit by candles; although in the real world (a loosely used term; Cambridge, and Oxford for that matter, are weird places slightly removed from the 'real world') the candles sit in candlesticks and don't float. Even though many of the colleges are medieval in age, their kitchens have kept up with the times, and now cater for all manner of dietary requests. At Wolfson, depending on what you indicated in the dietary requirements box when booking dinner, be it kosher or halal, nut-free or dairy-free, pescatarian or vegan, you get a little appropriately coloured card to place by your plate to alert the server. The gentleman seated across from me was a retired biochemist named Don, and he had just such a card. I asked him what that particular colour signalled.

'It means gluten-free,' Don said.

'But that's because Don has coeliac disease. It's not because he's being faddy,' his wife, Mary, who was sitting next to him chipped in. 'Ridiculous thing, going gluten-free for no good reason.'

I'd known Don and Mary a few years, and it's probably relevant to add that Mary was actually a wheat geneticist. A wheat geneticist married to a retired coeliac biochemist . . . I don't know why, but it amuses me every time I think of it.

Was Mary right, though? Is it absolutely ridiculous to be on a gluten-free diet if you are not a coeliac?

GLUTEN IS A PROTEIN AND NOT A CARB

A common misconception is that gluten is a type of carbohydrate. It isn't. It is actually a protein found in a number of grass-related grains such as wheat, barley, rye, oats and their various related species. More accurately, gluten is a composite of proteins termed prolamins and glutelins. In wheat, these are called gliadins and glutenin respectively. Gluten (from Latin *gluten* or 'glue') is 'activated' when flour meets water, and the resulting dough is kneaded. This activated gluten provides the characteristic of elasticity. It is why pizza dough can be whirled above one's head with abandon; it enables pasta to be rolled translucently thin while still holding together; it allows ramen and egg noodles to be stretched out long and skinny, ideal for slurping from a large bowl; and it captures the carbon dioxide produced by yeast-metabolising sugar to form millions of air bubbles, thus making bread rise. Gluten enables these and many other delicious foods, and that is a good thing.

Of course, gluten doesn't have to be 'activated' to find its way into food. Any food which uses wheat flour as a thickener for sauces and gravies, in batters, or as a light dusting to provide a little texture after pan frying, will contain gluten. Many traditional soy sauces include wheat in the fermentation process and so contain gluten (the exception being Japanese Tamari soy sauce, which is wheat-free and hence gluten-free). And because barley is the key grain used in brewing, most beers also contain gluten. In these recipes, the requirement for starch (a thickening agent) or sugars (for fermentation) are the reasons grains are used; gluten is simply a bystander.

COELIAC DISEASE

For people with coeliac disease, however, gluten is, without exaggeration, seriously bad news. Coeliac disease is an autoimmune disorder (when the body's immune system, for one reason or another, begins to attack itself) primarily affecting the small intestine. It is caused by the ingestion of gluten in genetically predisposed people, where it triggers an autoimmune attack on the gut. The

word 'coeliac' comes from the Greek κοιλιακός (koiliakos), meaning 'abdominal'. The 'classic' symptoms of coeliac disease include
chronic diarrhoea and abdominal distention, malabsorption, loss
of appetite, and impaired growth. Whilst it was initially thought
to be a disease that emerged primarily in small children younger
than two years of age, we now know that it can present at any
age, all the way into adulthood. Don, the retired biochemist from
Wolfson, for example, was not diagnosed till well past middle-age.
The condition affects approximately 1–2 per cent of the general
population, but many cases remain undiagnosed and untreated,
and these people are therefore at risk for serious long-term health
complications.[1] Untreated coeliac disease reduces quality of life,
and may result in iron deficiency, osteoporosis, an increased risk
of intestinal lymphomas (a type of cancer) and increased mortality.

Aretaeus, a second-century Greek physician, first coined the
term 'coeliac disease' to describe a malabsorptive syndrome with
chronic diarrhoea. However, it was the paediatrician Samuel Gee
who gave the first modern-day description of the condition. In
a lecture in 1887 at the Great Ormond Street Hospital for Sick
Children, London, Samuel presented cases of children with the
condition, acknowledging earlier descriptions of the disease, and
formalised the name 'coeliac'. Crucially, he was prescient in recog-
nising that, 'If the patient can be cured at all, it must be by means
of diet.' Samuel worked out, for example, that starchy foods should
be avoided and that milk intolerance became a problem (because
of all the damage to the intestinal lining). He never, however, made
the link to specific grains, so also excluded rice, as well as other
starchy vegetables, all of which don't contain gluten, from his prescribed diet. The linking of wheat to the disease was credited to the
Dutch paediatrician Dr Willem Karel Dicke in the 1940s, when he
noticed that the symptoms of his patients improved in the Dutch
'hunger winter' of 1944, during which flour was not available.[2] The
final leap was made by Charlotte Anderson and her colleagues in

Birmingham, England, in 1952,[3] who showed that it was specifically the gluten fraction of wheat flour (as opposed to the starch fraction) that was the triggering factor in coeliac disease.

The inner wall of a typical healthy small intestine is covered in millions of 'villi', which are tiny finger-like projections about 0.5–1 millimetre in size; just imagine a shag-pile carpet that has been rolled up into a tube, and you'd get a pretty good magnified idea of what it should look like. The villi act to increase the surface area through which the absorption of nutrients like sugars, fatty-acids and amino acids can occur. In addition, each villus has a good blood-supply and its surface is only one cell thick, which means that nutrients are absorbed easily and then rapidly carried away by the blood to other parts of the body. Interspersed amongst this single layer of absorptive cells are different 'enteroendocrine' cells, which secrete gut hormones in response to the presence of nutrients. This is the delicate environment that is under attack in coeliac disease. At its most severe, the villi actually disappear, and the internal lining of the small intestine becomes smooth and inflamed, which is most certainly undesirable.

When gluten is consumed and enters the gut, the gliadin component links up with a protein in the small intestine called 'tissue transglutaminase'. In certain susceptible people, this gliadin-transglutaminase complex triggers the production of auto-antibodies. Antibodies are part of the immune system, and one of their roles is normally to bind to proteins on an attacking virus or bacteria, for example, marking it out for destruction by immune cells. Auto-antibodies, however, recognise proteins from our own self, and you can see how that can go wrong pretty quickly. The reasons for the triggering of this autoimmune response have not been entirely worked out, but there are undoubtedly genetic influences, as well as a role for an increase in gut permeability or leakiness (this is a key point, which I will discuss in detail later). The bottom line is, because transglutaminase resides in the lining of the small intestine, when anti-transglutaminase auto-antibodies mark the protein out for destruction, the gut lining, with all its delicate villi, gets damaged as well, and *voilà*, we have coeliac disease.

Currently, the only available treatment for coeliac disease is sticking to a strict gluten-free diet. If you remove the gluten, the gut begins to heal. Unfortunately, if gluten is reintroduced, the body begins to attack the gut lining again, so coeliacs have to stay gluten-free for life. Adhering to such a diet can be difficult, however, owing to minute amounts of gluten that may be present on gluten-free foods. Depending on the severity of the disease, these trace amounts can be as harmful as lack of adherence to a gluten-free diet.

That being said, awareness, and therefore availability, of gluten-free food has never been higher. I once visited and filmed at Manna Dew, an artisanal bakery located in Battersea, south-west London. Manna Dew is owned and run by Mohamed Aboughazala, and is an entirely gluten-free establishment. You might have thought that a gluten-free bakery would not be the most promising of places to grab a sandwich, but Mohamed said to me:

'This is not a "gluten-free" bakery. This is a bakery that happens to be gluten-free.'

His aim was to create great bread in both taste and texture and people were not going to be able to tell that it was gluten-free. I was sceptical, but was prepared to be convinced, so I helped Mohamed make a batch of his famous olive oil focaccia (an Italian flatbread). The process was undoubtedly more complicated, and took more time than traditional bread, because it was gluten-free. However, the end product was extraordinary. I nicked a little piece just as it was warm out of the oven; the texture was fluffy and light, and it was wonderfully delicious. Mohamed was right, I could not tell that it was gluten-free. Manna Dew was initially set up because Mohamed saw a gap in the market for 'high-end' gluten-free bread, and most of his customers were indeed coeliacs.

As word has spread, now some of his customers have no issues with gluten at all and just happen to like the bread. However, his fastest-growing market are those who say that they are suffering from 'non-coeliac gluten sensitivity'.

GLUTEN SENSITIVITY

'Non-coeliac gluten sensitivity' is a term used to describe individuals who have a negative coeliac diagnosis, but have symptoms, intestinal or otherwise, related to ingestion of grains that contain gluten; critically, these symptoms improve or go away when the offending gluten is removed from their diet. The earliest descriptions that I could find of non-coeliac gluten sensitivity were in two papers published in the 1970s. The first was a 1976 paper by B. T. Cooper and colleagues in *Gut* entitled 'Proceedings: Chronic diarrhoea and gluten sensitivity,'[4] and the second was by A. Ellis and B. D. Linaker called, 'Non-coeliac gluten sensitivity?' published in *The Lancet* in 1978.[5] Then there was a long period of quiet, until it was 'rediscovered' in 2010 when Anna Sapone and Alessio Fasano published a paper describing the clinical and pathophysiological features of the condition.[6] The problem is, unlike coeliac disease, no specific biological markers have yet been identified and validated for non-coeliac gluten sensitivity. Currently, a gold-standard diagnosis of non-coeliac gluten sensitivity can really only be achieved with a 'double blind crossover' gluten challenge. 'Double blind' meaning that neither the physician nor the patient knows which is the placebo and which is the 'test' (only a third person, who blinded the test, knows); crossover meaning that the patient gets both the placebo and the test over two different periods. So in a blinded gluten challenge, a patient is given 8g of gluten (this approximates the amount found in two slices of bread) or placebo for 1 week each, separated by a 1-week gluten-free washout period to ensure no residual effects of the gluten test. Symptoms are then monitored throughout the challenge, providing a clear answer as to which, if any, have anything to do with the presence of gluten.

The problem is that such a blinded challenge can really only be undertaken in a research setting. It is simply not feasible in a typical clinical scenario, because it takes too long and is too labour-intensive. Thus, the frequency of 'true' non-coeliac gluten sensitivity is unknown, but it is estimated to be slightly more common than coeliac disease. As a result of this uncertainty, the number of papers reporting on non-coeliac gluten sensitivity, since the now seminal 2010 paper by Fasano, has grown exponentially, together with the number of persons treated with a gluten-free diet, because of a wide array of symptoms or conditions.

Another difficulty is that the symptoms of non-coeliac gluten sensitivity overlap with those of irritable bowel syndrome (IBS), which is far more common (10–15 per cent of the population), and include abdominal pain, gas, distension and irregular bowel movements. Additionally, extra-intestinal symptoms of non-coeliac gluten sensitivity (which overlap with coeliac disease) include headaches or migraine, foggy mind, chronic fatigue, joint and muscle pain, tingling of the extremities, leg or arm numbness, eczema, anaemia and depression. Just to be clear, someone with *bona fide* non-coeliac gluten sensitivity is not going to exhibit the entire list above; rather, the specific constellation of symptoms that present are going to depend entirely on the individual. The problem is the list is so broad, that all of us will have experienced at least one of the symptoms recently, or even right now! If we typed some combination of these symptoms into an internet search engine, gluten sensitivity (or multiple sclerosis, or fibromyalgia, or Lyme disease, or indeed IBS) would emerge as a possible diagnosis by Doctor Google. With no readily accessible test and a relatively simple solution of going gluten-free, it is very easy to see how many people end up self-diagnosing with gluten sensitivity.

In truth, as Fasano's paper was published in an academic journal, and very few people aside from other nerdy scientist folk (such as yours truly) read academic journals, if there had been no additional intervention, non-coeliac gluten sensitivity would have, in all likelihood, remained an academic curiosity. However, in 2011, a cardiologist from Milwaukee, Wisconsin, William (Bill) Davis, who clearly had taken at least some inspiration from Fasano, published a book entitled *Wheat Belly*. It became a runaway bestseller, with more than 2 million copies sold worldwide. In fact, *Wheat Belly* turned out to be one of the foundational texts that has fuelled (and continues to fan the flames of) the 'gluten-free' movement, elevating it from a niche diet for coeliacs to a *cause célèbre* embraced by the Hollywood glitterati, Instagram gurus and elite athletes alike.

A HAMBURGER WITH NO BUN

Late in 2016, I took a week-long trip to the United States with the BBC *Horizon* documentary team, to film a series of interviews for our investigative piece into 'clean-eating'. After the visit with Robert Young at his pH Miracle Ranch in California (more on this later), we travelled to Cleveland, Ohio; home to Superman, the Cleveland Browns (American) football team and the Rock & Roll Hall of Fame. About an hour's drive south of the city, we found ourselves in the small rural Ohioan town of Lodi. It was smack bang in the middle of Nowhere, Nowhere, and the most notable thing about the town was that it gave its name to the nearby community of over 2,000 'Lodi Amish'. On Bank Street, across the road from the railway tracks and right next to a gas station, was a restaurant-diner called 'Cruisers', where I had organised to meet up with Bill Davis. Just as Bill drove up, two horse and buggies went clip-clopping past, their Amish passengers, in traditional dress, headed to the gas station to pick up fuel.

When Bill and I entered the diner, it felt as if we were stepping back in time to the 1950s, replete with red and chrome stools by the bar, red faux-leather upholstered seats in the booths and a gum-chewing waitress called Alice (she was not actually called Alice, but she could have been). Bill and I found a booth and sat down.

Bill Davis sets out his stall very early in *Wheat Belly*. In the introduction, he says:

'I am going to argue that the problem with the diet and health of most Americans is not fat, not sugar . . . not the demise of the agrarian lifestyle; it's WHEAT – or what we are being sold that is called wheat.' [7]

This is pretty much the *'haiku'* synopsis of the book. Bill blames wheat for much, if not all, of our dietary ills and also argues that these problems have been exacerbated because the wheat we eat today is 'not really wheat at all but the transformed product of genetic research'. But the real reason why so many find his message attractive is because he absolves blame from fat and sugar, and everything else actually. The jacket cover of his book reads:

'The effortless health and weight-loss solution; No exercise, no calorie counting, no denial.'

Eat as much of what you want, just give up wheat, and all your health problems will disappear? What's not to like? Sign me up!

(Spoiler alert: Absolute statements in science are very rarely correct. But I will deploy one now; anybody who is trying to sell you an *effortless* weight-loss solution is simply not telling the truth.)

The other classic strategy employed by Bill is to gain the empathy of the reader by sharing his personal story early in Chapter 1; how he battled with his weight for much of his life, and was diagnosed with type 2 diabetes when he was about forty years old. As Bill tells it, his 'Damascene conversion' occurred when he caught sight of himself in a beach-holiday snap taken by his wife. Through personal trial and error, he worked out that by cutting out wheat, his weight fell away, and with it his diabetes. It was then that he began his war on wheat and, ultimately, his war on ALL grains.

As I looked across the table to Bill Davis, now in his mid-fifties, he did look in great shape!

'I asked my many patients, "remove grains and sugars, let's see what happens".'

He then gave me multiple examples of his patients' improvement in metabolic health: lowering of LDL (Low-density lipoprotein – these transfer cholesterol and fat around the body); reversal of diabetes; and crucially, tremendous weight loss.

As we were chatting, 'Alice' came up to take our order.

'ALICE'   Are you ready to order, or do you need a few minutes?

BILL   I'm OK.

ME   You're, you're OK? Really?

BILL   I'll just, I'll just have, uh, how about a hamburger with no bun?

'ALICE'   A hamburger with no bun . . .

BILL   Without a bun.

'ALICE'   uhuh . . .

I ordered French toast with bacon and maple syrup. I'm sure Bill was horrified, but he was simply too polite to say anything.

FRANKENWHEAT

Bill's first big argument is that the ubiquitous dwarf wheat we eat today is nothing like the tall ancestral wheat that grew on the prairie under big skies, inspiring the opening lyric from 'America the Beautiful':

'O beautiful for spacious skies; For amber waves of grain.'[8]

Bill argues that today's wheat has been so heavily genetically modified by hybridisation and breeding that it is no longer 'natural' but has become 'synthetic'; and it is this synthetic 'Frankenwheat' that is causing all of our diet-related illnesses. This all sounds very scary, and a quick glance online reveals that many people are buying this argument. There is, dare I say, an almost 'hipster'-like movement towards ancient or heritage wheats like Einkorn, because they are perceived to be healthier (they certainly taste different) than our modern wheat *Triticum aestivum*.

If you would permit me, a very brief wheat-genetics primer. Ancestral wheat used to be 'diploid', which meant they had two copies of every gene. Einkorn is an example of a 'diploid' wheat. The vast majority of mammals, including us humans, are diploid; one copy of each gene from our mother and the other copy from our father. Half a million years ago, two diploid wheat ancestors merged together to form a 'tetraploid' plant. This new wheat species now had four copies of each gene. This process of increasing gene copies is known as 'polyploidy', which is very common in plants. Emmer wheat for example, is tetraploid. Then approximately 8,000 years ago, a tetraploid wheat was hybridised with another diploid wheat to give our modern hexaploid (6 copies of each gene) wheat, *Triticum aestivum*. All of our different modern strains of wheat have been bred or hybridised from *Triticum aestivum*.[9] The reason I go into this is because Bill hijacks this information and uses it to construct his 'Frankenwheat' argument.

When you are breeding a plant, you do it from the same strain, but may choose different characteristics to select for, such as height or size of seed. When you are hybridising a plant, you may pick two strains with very different characteristics; one may be very short and another may have very large seeds that fall off easily. You would cross these in the hope of getting a plant that is both short and has large seeds that easily fall off, and you may or may not be successful. Once you find a desirable trait from hybridisation, you can then fix the trait into the strain by breeding.

So let's set some facts straight. Hybridised wheat is NOT genetically modified (GM) wheat. At the time of writing, there is no commercially available GM wheat in the food chain. None. Hybridisation is a traditional plant-breeding technique and there is therefore nothing 'synthetic' about it. The approach of trait selection in breeding has been used by farmers since the dawn of agriculture, as I discuss in Chapter 4, for every plant and animal that we have ever domesticated. The only difference is while in the past we would be assessing the characteristics by sight and feel, today we have the molecular tools to understand (or try and understand) the genetic changes underlying many of the traits.

Bill is right that 99 per cent of the wheat grown today is dwarf wheat. Tall wheat would grow to 4 feet (1.2 metres) high, whereas today's shorter variety reaches half that height. Because the seeds appear near the top of the plant, short wheat takes less energy and less time to grow (2 feet or 0.6 metres of strawless energy!) before it begins to produce seeds. The other problem with tall wheat is that it is wavy and very top-heavy once the seeds are at full size, resulting in a percentage of wheat flopping over, with the seeds getting stuck in the ground and not being harvested. This is far less likely to happen with the shorter variety. Thus, dwarf wheat, which was hybridised and bred in Mexico by Norman Borlaug in the mid-1940s–50s, required fewer resources to produce the same amount of food. This was such a critical development in increasing the world's food supply on a planet rapidly becoming more crowded that Norman was awarded the Nobel Peace Prize in 1970.

But Bill then goes on to question the safety of the dwarf wheat that all of us eat today. He claims that hybridisation could generate plants that are unsafe for consumption, with the process creating up to 5 per cent of proteins that are unique and not seen in either parent, some of which have potentially toxic effects. Stop it, please. Because proteins are assembled based on the instructions carried in genes, the only way for 'new' or 'unique' proteins to be made is if the DNA sequence of the genes has been mutated or changed. Hybridisation, however, relies on the mixing of genes, and therefore proteins, that are already present in the parent plants, in order to produce new characteristics. It does not, CANNOT, result in new proteins.

IT DOESN'T MAKE MONEY

Since 2011, Bill has expanded his war on wheat to now include ALL grains, claiming, with fervent belief, that humans were never meant to eat grain. This is the same claim made by the Paleo movement, which I tackled in Chapter 4. Bill's second big argument, however, is that grains are the cause of many diseases, including an assortment of neurological disorders such as schizophrenia, eczema, type 2 diabetes and heart disease. If that wasn't enough, he also places the blame of ALL autoimmune conditions, such as coeliac disease, rheumatoid arthritis and type 1 diabetes, on grains. But what Bill undoubtedly sees as the biggest problem is that it is wheat in particular that has made us fat. He writes in the introduction to *Wheat Belly*, 'Extraordinary as these results may sound, there is ample scientific research to implicate wheat as a root cause of these conditions – and to indicate that removal of wheat can reduce or relieve symptoms entirely ... many of the lessons I've learnt were demonstrated in clinical studies decades ago ... I've simply put two and two together ...'[10]

I asked Bill why, if ample scientific data was available as he claimed, had other scientists or health professionals not put two and two together as well? He replied:

'I'll give you a very cynical view; it doesn't make money.'

Aha. Of course.

This is the pervasive conspiracy theory that the medical profession are in cahoots with 'big pharma' to make *beaucoup* bucks selling pills, and so have no reason, or worse, don't want, to see a dietary approach to reversing illness work. Bill is by no means unique in taking this view, as you will see in the following chapters. Are the pharmaceutical industry trying to make money? Of course they are! They are, after all, companies with costs, employees and shareholders to keep happy. But, here's the thing that many people forget; they only make money if what they sell *works* and people get *better*. The whole idea that most doctors, nurses, scientists and other health professionals today are 'in the pocket of big pharma' and want to see people remain unhealthy at the expense of pushing pills is, to be frank, ludicrous.

First, most of the medical profession are not paid by pharma; rather, they are employed by hospitals or universities or, here in the UK, by the National Health Service (NHS), to try and help people get better. In the UK, for example, because of the NHS, doctors do not have any financial incentive to prescribe one treatment over another. In fact, the NHS is under such constant financial pressure to find the most economical solution to all problems that if there was a genuine dietary treatment option that worked for a particular disease, they would use it. Second, pharma do indeed fund academics and clinicians to undertake studies and trials, which in this day and age have to be declared in any resulting publications and presentations. Does this constitute 'influence'? I don't think so. Unlike in academia, there is little pressure to 'publish or perish' in the pharma industry. The principal pieces of data that the industry want from any funded study is whether a treatment works or not, and if it works, are there any significant side-effects. Today, if some potential drug or compound doesn't work, or has the potential to cause more harm than good, it will be pulled faster than you can say *'Boo'*, because anything bad that happens has the potential to bring a company down. So even putting aside ethics and morals, it makes absolutely no financial sense to influence results one way or the other.

WHEAT BELLY

The widespread use of vertically challenged wheat in agriculture over the past few decades happened to coincide with our increasing waistlines; however, the leap taking Bill from this correlation to wheat height being a causative factor in obesity is a very large one. A multitude of other changes are also correlated with the increasing rates of obesity, including the dramatic drop in our daily physical activity, our increased accessibility to food, the drop in the cost of food, as well as changes in the type of food that we eat. Is it going to be any one specific change, such as a predilection for wheat-based food products, which has made us become more obese? Highly unlikely. It makes far more sense that a shift in the environment as a whole has led to a collective increase in our waistlines.

Bill's choice of title for his book is also very interesting. He hasn't called it 'Wheat Derrière' or 'Thighs of Wheat' or 'Wheat Wobble' or 'Wheat-any-other-body-part'. Bill purposefully used 'Belly' because he believed that the consumption of wheat leads to a build-up, specifically, of visceral fat. As I've discussed, visceral fat is stored around the organs and tends to result in a large but tight belly, the stereotypical 'beer-belly', hence Bill's use of 'Wheat-belly'. This is in contrast to 'subcutaneous fat', which sits just under the skin and can therefore accumulate anywhere. It is true that visceral fat is worse for your health than fat anywhere else in your body, and is linked to a higher risk of insulin resistance and diabetes, as well as an increased the risk of strokes, heart disease and some cancers. Bill's belief that wheat causes increased amounts of visceral fat leads him to link all of these diseases to wheat.

However, as we've seen, it is clear that while you can do something about how MUCH fat you are carrying, you actually have no control over WHERE you put your fat, which is almost entirely down to your genes.[11] Will eating too much pasta or bread or couscous lead you to gain weight? Undoubtedly so. Will excess wheat-based calories be shunted directly to toxic visceral fat, thereby leading to an early grave? That very much depends on your own personal biology; your sex, for example, has an enormous influence, with men more likely to have a higher store of visceral fat than women. But crucially, even if you were more likely to gain visceral fat than someone else, there is no evidence that eating too much wheat is any worse than having too much sugar or fat or anything else for that matter.

DOES A GLUTEN-FREE DIET REVERSE DISEASE?

A rhetorical strategy employed by Bill to great effect is the use of anecdote and testimonials to support his arguments. Here is an example *pro forma* anecdote:

'Mrs Smith came to me with disease X and symptom Y; I prescribed a strict gluten-free diet, and six months later Mrs Smith came back leaner and meaner and with miraculous improvement of disease X and no more symptom Y. Hooray gluten-free!'

There are two main problems with using anecdote as primary evidence. First, it is uncontrolled. How do we know it was the removal of wheat *per se*, rather than a change in something else? Because you tend to go to the doctor when you are feeling really bad, how do we know that Mrs Smith wasn't going to get better anyway, with or without the removal of wheat? Second, even if the removal of wheat helped Mrs Smith feel better, how do we know whether everyone else is going to respond in the same way?

Compare this to the 'double blind crossover' gluten challenge that I discuss above, which is controlled for compliance and specificity of treatment, and removes bias from either the patient or the physician from the equation, thus giving you confidence in the validity of the results.

A gluten-free diet, however, does appear to be effective in certain aspects of health. In particular, if you analyse the anecdotes that Bill has chosen to use as a whole, there appears to be a consistent effect of tremendous weight loss, with some patients losing up to 30 kilograms. With multiple anecdotes giving the same effect, surely this is something approaching evidence of a gluten-free diet having a positive effect? I would agree with this assessment. What is less clear, however, is what elements of the gluten-free diet are responsible for mediating the weight loss. In North America and Europe, because wheat and rye are such a ubiquitous source of carbohydrates, a gluten-free diet essentially means a pretty restrictive low-carb diet. Bill actually suggests that the Atkins Diet works because of the removal of gluten, rather than the fact that it is low in carbohydrates. In fact, with Bill actively encouraging eating as much meat and fat as one would like, in conjunction with removing gluten-containing grains, what you actually end up with is a 'low-carb, high-protein' diet. And as we know from Chapter 4, high-protein diets do indeed work, at least in the short term, for weight loss. In a higher protein diet, because proteins are less calorically available and take longer to digest than fat and carbs, they end up travelling further down the gut, releasing hormones that make you feel fuller. Feeling fuller means you eat less, which is still the most effective way to lose weight. So a gluten-free diet is effective in the short term for weight loss, not because of the removal of gluten, but because it creates a calorie deficit, through a combination of a low-carbohydrate restrictive diet coupled with increased protein.

What about all the other illnesses that Bill blames on wheat?

Because many other diseases including type 2 diabetes, heart disease, certain cancers and also neurological disorders such as Alzheimer's are linked to obesity, losing a large amount of weight reverses type 2 diabetes in most (but not all) people and reduces the risk for all the other diseases. Thus, the most likely explanation for the miraculous health improvements that Bill Davis sees in his patients after they go on a gluten-free diet is because they lose large amounts of weight, rather than because of the removal of gluten *per se*.

IS GLUTEN HARMFUL FOR EVERYONE?

What surprised me the most from my meeting with Bill Davis, however, was his strong belief that gluten was harmful to ALL of us, to one degree or another. At this point in the interview, we had moved from the restaurant to a wheat farm; the BBC do like a sense of space! The problem was, it was a late rainy September day and the harvest was already in, so we were essentially standing in a muddy field, surrounded by grain silos and farm equipment, and getting soggy. Perhaps it was a fitting place, after all, to be speaking with an anti-wheat evangelist!

To support his contention that gluten is harmful to everyone, Bill tells me of the work of Dr Alessio Fasano.

Originally from Naples in Italy, Dr Alessio Fasano is now based at the Centre for Coeliac Research, Massachusetts General Hospital, Boston, and is one of the world's leading experts in coeliac disease and the role of gluten in health and disease. In 2003, Fasano discovered that coeliac disease, far from being a very rare early childhood disease, representing maybe 2/10,000 live births, can actually emerge at any age and affects around 1 per cent of the population.[12] Then in 2010, as I discussed earlier, he 'rediscovered' non-coeliac gluten sensitivity.[13]

The Fasano lab has also shown that gluten (specifically the gliadin component) initiates the steps that can create gut leakiness or intestinal permeability,[14] by triggering the release of a rather alien-sounding protein called zonulin. Zonulin, as it turns out, is a master regulator of intestinal permeability.[15] The key function of the gastrointestinal tract is to digest food, absorb as much of the nutrients and water as possible, and then get rid of all of the waste products in preparation for your next meal; it is your 'food to poop tube'. As a result, the intestinal lining has to thread a fine line, making sure that vital nutrients are allowed through, while keeping bacteria, potential toxins and anything else destined for the poop end of the tube, out of the blood supply. This protective layer, particularly in the small intestine, is only one cell thick. These cells work very hard and are replaced every few days. These intestinal cells are 'polarised', meaning that they are directional, with different functions at either end. One end of the cell points into the actual gut tube (known as the lumen), sensing and absorbing nutrients as they pass by, while the other end of the cell is in contact with the blood supply, allowing absorbed nutrients and any secreted hormones to be transported efficiently away. Fasano has shown that zonulin, which comes from the Latin *zonula* for small belt or girdle, regulates the permeability of that protective single cell layer lining the intestine. If too much zonulin is produced, however, the gut goes from being permeable in a controlled fashion, to being leaky, which by definition is uncontrolled. This means, of course, that some of the stuff you are trying to keep out of the blood supply is now coming in. Bill's interpretation of this data is that gluten triggers the release of zonulin, increasing gut leakiness, allowing in all types of nasty bugs and toxins, and thus is the first step in generating autoimmune diseases. Hence Bill's contention that gluten is the cause of all autoimmune disease.

OK, just hang on. Before all of you go running to the kitchen to throw out your bread and pasta, I would just like to clarify that

I am not talking about perforations, gaping holes or a ruptured gut, which you would know about as it results, pretty acutely, in death. Rather I'm speaking of leakiness at the molecular level, where slightly larger compounds that are normally kept out are now being let in. In some people, this increased permeability, this leakiness, is indeed a precursor to autoimmune conditions and chronic inflammatory diseases, including coeliac disease. So Bill is partially correct. The problem is, he has extrapolated these findings to mean that all of our guts are being turned into sieves whenever we eat wheat.

After our trip to Ohio, we then headed to Boston to interview Dr Fasano. When Bill's argument, that the ingestion of gluten harms everybody, was put to Fasano, he was the paragon of diplomacy:

'I respect and like some of the aspects of Dr Davis, so it's not that I'm an enemy. Of course, I'd be ecstatic if he's right; but honestly I don't think that is the case.'

First of all, gluten doesn't increase zonulin levels in everyone. Second, in his latest experiment, Fasano and his team have genetically engineered mice to produce too much zonulin, and show that under normal conditions, these mice are no different from regular 'wild-type' mice. It is only when both strains of mice are stressed with a toxin that differences are seen; with the mice producing too much zonulin becoming ill and nothing happening to the 'wild-type' mice.[16] In other words, just having too much zonulin, and therefore a leaky gut, in and of itself is not enough to cause disease. These are, of course, animal studies, and one has to be careful with extending any interpretation directly to humans. But this is just one study of many conducted by Fasano and others over the past few years on the role of gluten in causing disease. Fasano has concluded that gluten is only harmful in conjunction with four other problems – a genetic predisposition, a leaky gut (through increased zonulin), a faulty immune system *and* imbalanced gut microbes.

To date, there is no evidence that supports what Bill Davis believes, that consuming gluten causes harm to everyone without exception.

FODMAPS

As I mention previously, one of the difficulties of diagnosing non-coeliac gluten sensitivity is that the symptoms overlap with those of irritable bowel syndrome (IBS), which is far more common (10-15 per cent of the population), and include abdominal pain, gas, distension and irregular bowel movements. Numerous studies show that the majority of patients with IBS (70 per cent–89 per cent) report that specific foods, such as ingestion of certain carbohydrates, can lead to exacerbation of gastrointestinal symptoms. In 2005, Peter Gibson and Susan Shepherd from Monash University in Melbourne, Australia, proposed that excessive consumption of 'fermentable oligosaccharides, disaccharides, and monosaccharides and polyols' or FODMAPs, increased susceptibility to Crohn's Disease.[17] Crohn's is an inflammatory bowel disorder, and it is certainly a far more severe condition than IBS. However, a few years later, in 2010, Gibson and Shepherd together with other colleagues linked high levels of FODMAPs to IBS as well.[18]

So what are FODMAPs exactly? Well, saccharides is another word for carbohydrates. Glucose is a monosaccharide; sucrose, which is formed of one glucose and one fructose molecule, is a disaccharide; oligosaccharides are short strings of saccharides three to ten molecules in length; while polyols are sugar 'alcohols' – hence the 'ols' at the end of the word. But not all saccharides are FODMAPs. FODMAPs are, by their nature, (relatively) poorly absorbed and so get to the lower small or upper large intestine. Once they get to that region of the gut, they then have to be fermentable by the bacteria that are present there. Glucose is very easily absorbed and so doesn't hang about to be fermented; while cellulose, which is what makes up the fibre in plants, we cannot digest or ferment, so goes right through us (like sweetcorn or celery).

All mammals, including humans, have an entire ecosystem of trillions of bacteria that live symbiotically in our gut. They perform a multitude of tasks, in particular shaping our immune systems and influencing our metabolism and our ability to absorb nutrients. There is a famous (scientific) urban myth that there are more bacterial denizens in our gut than we have cells in our body. This, as it turns out, is not true; there are probably the same number of bacteria in us as we have cells . . . which still number in the trillions and is a pretty amazing fact! In some mammals, the gut bacteria play such a crucial role in digestion that entire new organs have evolved to house them. Like humans, most mammals are unable to digest cellulose. Ruminants, however, which include cows, sheep, goats and horses, have an entirely separate compartment in their digestive system call the rumen, where bacteria are able to ferment cellulose, found in grass and leaves for instance, thereby making the calories available for use. Humans do not have a rumen, but our own personalised population of microorganisms do ferment some of the ingested carbohydrates, producing gas as one of the by-products, as anyone that has just eaten a whole heap of beans or Brussels sprouts can attest. It just so happens that beans contain high amounts of FODMAPs.

The main monosaccharide FODMAP is fructose. This carbohydrate is a sugar and is present in many fruits as well as honey. While glucose is universally easily absorbed, the same is not true for fructose. We all differ in the way our gut absorbs fructose, with some people very good at absorbing it and others not so good. It is when the amount of fructose exceeds the amount of glucose that problems start to occur. The major FODMAP disaccharide is lactose, which is formed of one molecule of galactose and one of glucose; this sugar is found primarily in dairy products and, like fructose, there is a large biological variation in how effectively, or whether we can at all, metabolise and absorb lactose. All oligosaccharides are considered FODMAPs, and dietary sources include wheat, legumes and other vegetables such as onion and garlic. Most, if not all, polyols would be considered FODMAPs, and are, today, found in various diet and sugar-free foods to lower their calorific content. Examples of polyols are sorbitol and xylitol.

In people with IBS, foods high in FODMAPs are thought to cause problems in three different ways.[19] The first is through a build-up of water. When there is a higher concentration of sugars such as fructose and/or lactose in the gut due to poor absorption, osmosis drives water in to the space to try and dilute out the sugar. This increased volume of the gut can cause discomfort in some and pain in others, and also result in diarrhoea. The second is through the build-up of gas through fermentation of the higher concentrations of FODMAPs. The gas, like water, can cause pain and discomfort in those who are hypersensitive to the distension. Finally, it is thought that FODMAPs can cause a change in the bacterial flora, so-called dysbiosis. This in turn can trigger gut inflammation, pain and increased gut permeability.

As I have mentioned, these symptoms of IBS overlap with that seen in non-coeliac gluten intolerance, and gluten-containing cereals, particularly wheat, are a primary source of FODMAPs. As a result, going on a gluten-free diet has the consequence of reducing the amount of FODMAPs being consumed. This may explain, at least in part, why some patients affected with irritable bowel symptoms may report a reduction of their symptoms after switching to a gluten-free diet.

GRAIN FREE

It is not entirely clear to me when the gluten-free movement began to take on elements of Paleo, evolving into 'grain-free'; but increasing numbers of people are now beginning to cut out all grains from their diet. The reasons are varied. Bill Davis, in *Wheat Belly*, says, 'Be gluten-free, but don't eat gluten-free.'[20] What he means is that swapping out wheat for another source of carbohydrates isn't more healthy and doesn't reduce calories; in fact it might actually be more unhealthy! I have to say that while I agree with Bill on this point, I'm also slightly confused. Doesn't taking this stance contradict his primary argument that wheat is the root of all evil? Anyway, if you visit Bill's website, you will see that he has now graduated from shunning wheat to shunning all grains.

The American neurologist David Perlmutter has written an anti-grain manifesto entitled *Grain Brain*. In it, he first endorses Bill Davis, agreeing entirely with the *Wheat Belly* message. He then takes things a whole lot further, turning his guns on the effect that grains have on the brain. Perlmutter blames everything found in grain – the gluten, complex carbohydrates and sugars – for causing brain diseases, especially Alzheimer's. He also trots out the same argument used by Bill with regards to 'Big Pharma':

'. . . is it that pharmaceutical companies are invested in discouraging the idea that lifestyle choices have a profound influence on brain health? Fair warning: I'm not going to have kind things to say about our pharmaceutical industry.'[21]

Thanks for the fair warning, Dave, it is appreciated. But extraordinarily, he then includes a myriad of other brain conditions as well; including migraines, depression, epilepsy, Tourette's, schizophrenia and other psychiatric disorders; all of which he claims are diseases of grains. What I do know is that type 2 diabetes is a risk factor for Alzheimer's, but we still do not know the underlying mechanism. Because eating too much of anything, including grains, leads to obesity, which is a major risk factor for type 2 diabetes, Perlmutter makes a huge leap to blame Alzheimer's and other brain disorders on grains. This is once again the correlation versus causation conundrum, and to date, there is no evidence that grains are what links type 2 diabetes and brain disorders. What is clear is that grain-free diets really are very restrictive, very low in carbohydrates, much more so than gluten-free diets. Perlmutter recommends eating as much meat and fat as one would like. So grain-free is very effective in the short term for weight loss because, like gluten-free, it creates a calorie deficit, through a combination of a low-carbohydrate restrictive diet coupled with increased protein. Weight loss results in a dramatically reduced risk of type 2 diabetes, and in turn a reduced risk of Alzheimer's.

WHY DOES THIS MATTER?

While we were standing in that muddy field in Ohio, I challenged Bill Davis about where his proof was that cutting out gluten would be the panacea for disease. I got a very interesting answer.

'The bar to prove, let's say, a new surgery is effective should be very high, you need very clear-cut data. If I were to say, let's eliminate watermelon from your diet, how confident do you have to be in order to do that? Well you could just try it, right? Nothing lost, nothing gained.'

In essence, I just got him to admit, on camera, that he didn't have the proof, that he didn't have clear-cut data. What Bill had done was to pull together a series of correlations, and then construct a theory around gluten.

Why does any of this matter, I hear you ask? If gluten-free diets, as I acknowledge, are effective for weight loss in some people, why does it matter how it works, as long as people become healthier?

Let's just imagine a situation where someone had self-diagnosed with non-coeliac gluten sensitivity, put themselves on a gluten-free regime, and then felt better. However, in reality, they had IBS, and the reason they felt better was because going gluten-free had reduced the FODMAPs in their diet. What then happens if they then decided to replace the wheat in their diet with beans, say, which happen to be high in FODMAPs? Their IBS symptoms would return, and they would not know why. The bottom line is that self-diagnosis should be discouraged. You have to know what is actually causing the symptoms, in order to avoid misdiagnosis and inappropriate treatment.

GOOD GLUTEN, BAD GLUTEN AND UGLY GLUTEN

One per cent of humans are coeliac, and an estimated 3–4 per cent are sensitive to gluten to some degree. Yet 25 per cent of us buy explicitly labelled gluten-free products, because we think it is somehow healthier, even if there is no scientific evidence to suggest that this is actually the case. Gluten-free has become such a selling point that manufacturers are now labelling things gluten-free that never contained gluten in the first place. Gluten-free rice, gluten-free corn, even gluten-free water. Most ridiculous of all is that inedible products are being marketed as gluten-free as well. There are, for example, hundreds of different gluten-free shampoos to suit all tastes. Type in 'gluten-free shampoo' into Google, and you will get more than six million hits! Some people argue that if you are a coeliac, then you need to use gluten-free shampoo, lest the gluten seeps through your skin. Not true. Please save your money. Gluten can only cause problems for coeliacs if it is ingested.

Are gluten-free products bad for us *per se*? No. But when you remove gluten, you need to replace it with something else that can do a similar job. Hence, gluten-free food can, in many situations contain more salt, or sugar, or fat, or require more processing. As a result, it also often costs more. But the crucial point is that gluten-free doesn't equate to healthy. In fact, to the contrary, scientists have shown that the avoidance of gluten may result in reduced consumption of beneficial whole grains, which may actually end up affecting cardiovascular risk.[22] Why might this be? Aside from a host of vitamins and nutrients, whole grains contain a large dose of fibre. Sufficient fibre in the diet is, of course, important for gut health, keeping everything at the poop end of the tube 'shipshape' and regular. It also does two other crucial things. First, it lowers the caloric availability of food by slowing the digestion and absorption of sugar and fat by the gut. Second, because it slows down digestion, food containing fibre travels farther down the gut, thus making you feel fuller. Of course other foods, such as fruit and vegetables, contain fibre. Yet a large part of society are still not consuming enough fibre. By all means, we need to have a sensible discussion about limiting our consumption of refined carbohydrates, such as white flour, which has had much of its fibre stripped out. Why on earth, however, would you want to remove whole grains, such an important source of fibre, from your diet?

So in conclusion, if you can't eat gluten, for heaven's sake, stay away from the stuff. If you can eat gluten, eat gluten. Because, please remember, a gluten-free doughnut is, after all, still a doughnut.

CHAPTER 6

Blessed are the cheesemakers

'Blessed are the cheesemakers!'
'What's so special about the cheesemakers?'
'Well, obviously it's not meant to be taken literally. It
refers to any manufacturer of dairy products.'

Monty Python's *Life of Brian* (1979)

My parents are ethnically Chinese and were born and raised in Singapore. But my dad, now retired, was a physician and an academic, and was always moving about for work or training purposes. He was doing his diabetes speciality training in 1973 at King's College Hospital, London, when I popped into the world. We then bounced about between Singapore, Boston, Singapore again and then San Francisco, before I eventually ended up here in Cambridge, UK more than two decades ago. However, of the many moves in my life, the one which resulted in the biggest culture shock for me was when we emigrated from Singapore to San Francisco in 1988. Prior to this, I was simply too young to know or, frankly, to care. Whereas when we moved to San Francisco, I had just turned fifteen years old and was therefore at the height of my monosyllabic teenaged-ness; when any change, even shifting where I was sitting in class, would have been considered a major upheaval. If that wasn't difficult enough, I made the move across the Pacific by myself, about three months ahead of my family, staying with one of my dad's brothers, so that I could catch the beginning of the school term. Everything about those first few months has been burnt into my psyche. To this day, I can still almost feel the chill of that first San Francisco evening as I walked wide-eyed out of the airport, a world away from the tropical heat and oppressive humidity of Singapore. I remembered my initial experience of the fog that rolled in on most summer evenings, blanketing the bay, with only the tops of the Golden Gate Bridge visible. The fog, in fact, is such a regular presence that it has acquired a name; known locally as 'Karl', it even has its own Twitter account, *@KarlTheFog*, for those interested in Bay Area meteorology and other fabulously foggy facts. Northern Californians are also a laid-back and friendly bunch, far more tactile and huggy than I was used to at the time. But above all, I vividly remember my initial encounters with American food (Californian food, more accurately), keeping in mind that this was the late 80s, when globalisation was not the all-encompassing force it is today. There was of course the portion sizes, which to be fair still shocks me when I find myself Stateside today; but there was also the large quantity of dairy products, particularly cheese, that was used in food, certainly when compared to 1980s Singapore.

My uncle, who I lived with in his downtown apartment during those first few months, was, shall we say, quite *laissez-faire* in his style of guardianship; which I am forever grateful for and still benefit from to this day. So before the closer eyes of the rest of my family joined me (keeping in mind that I was a hungry fifteen-year-old with a typically bottomless pit for a stomach), I experienced for the first time in my life: chilli with cheese, chilli-cheese-dogs, nachos with cheese, mac & cheese, cheese quesadillas, cheesy crab dip, cheesecake of all different varieties and Chicago-style deep dish pizza, amongst other culinary delights. I know it is difficult to believe, but I had not had any of these cheesy offerings prior to moving to San Francisco. It's not to say that some of these dishes would not have been available in Singapore, or in Boston where we lived when I was nine to ten years old; rather, my father simply would not have ordered them. My dad, you see, is, like the majority of Chinese folk, lactose intolerant. I did not know it then, but I am too.

Like going gluten-free, going dairy-free is *à la mode*, so I'm going to look at whether we should do so or not.

LACTOSE

Lactose is the primary sugar found in dairy products. It is a disaccharide, formed of one molecule each of the monosaccharides glucose and galactose. Humans, however, cannot absorb lactose. In order for us to use the energy locked up in the sugar, the small intestine produces an enzyme called lactase-phlorizin-hydrolase, or simply 'lactase', which breaks down lactose into its two simpler forms, glucose and galactose. The body then easily absorbs these simpler sugars into the bloodstream.

Although the inability to drink and eat dairy products (or more specifically, the inability to digest lactose) is commonly called 'lactose intolerance', this is actually somewhat of a misnomer. All human infants, all very young mammals actually, drink milk as the major energy source and are therefore lactose tolerant in early life; this is what defines us as mammals after all. Most humans then become increasingly lactose intolerant in the transition to adulthood. This is caused when the lactase in the small intestine gradually disappears, and as a consequence, lactose is no longer able to be digested. What then happens is the undigested lactose moves down from the small to the large intestine. Normally, in the lower part of the large intestine known as the colon, water is absorbed from whatever food remains are left after all the digestion and nutrient absorption further up in the small intestine. This changes it from a liquid to a solid form, leaving what is colloquially known as 'poop' (other four-letter words do exist, but this is a family-friendly book) or scientifically referred to as faeces. If, however, a large amount of undigested lactose makes it into the colon, two things happen; first, less water is absorbed by the gut, causing the faeces to be less solid or not solid at all; and second, the bacteria that reside in the colon begins to ferment the lactose, producing gas. This results in the characteristic digestive symptoms of lactose intolerance, which include abdominal bloating (a feeling of uncomfortable fullness in the abdomen), often leading to abdominal pain, diarrhoea, gas and sometimes nausea. These unpleasant effects typically occur in lactose-intolerant individuals, between 30 minutes to two hours after consuming milk or milk products. Symptoms can range from mild to severe depending on the amount of lactose that has been consumed and also the amount a person can tolerate (more about this later).

However, in many people, the lactase levels in their small intestine do not decrease with age, and as a result they are able to digest lactose all through life. This is known as 'lactase persistence', a characteristic shared by about 35 per cent of adult humans, particularly those of Northern European ancestry, as well as pockets of smaller populations in Africa and Northern India.[1]

So why have some populations adapted to consume dairy products when others have not?

INTOLERANCE IS NOT AN ALLERGY

Before answering this question, I do think it is important to clear up a common misconception. Being intolerant of lactose is a completely different thing from having a milk allergy. Intolerance is a result of the inability to digest the sugar present in milk; it is a biochemical problem emerging from an enzyme deficiency.

An allergy, however, is having an adverse immune response to the protein in milk. Milk allergies are usually observed in infants and young children, affecting between 2 and 3 per cent of infants. The symptoms for a milk allergy are common to many other allergies, and can include hives and swelling, vomiting and wheezing. In rare circumstances, it can cause anaphylaxis (in about 1–2 per cent of cases), which is a severe, life-threatening allergic reaction. However, milk allergy often disappears with age, usually during early childhood, or at the latest by the time of adolescence.[2]

But just to enunciate this critical point again, *intolerance is NOT an allergy.*

THE DAWN OF DAIRYING

Back to the matter at hand. To answer the question, let's first look at how we came to drink and eat dairy in the first place. The agricultural revolution encompassed not only the cultivation of plants, but also the domestication of large mammals. This began some 1,500 years after the first crops were farmed, starting with sheep about 10,500 years ago, and goats 10,000 years ago, both in and around what is now Turkey.[3] Cattle were then domesticated 9,000 years ago in the Eastern Sahara.[4] These animals would have been initially kept for meat, their skin, their wool (if they were a sheep), their sinew and any other useful bits. This was probably the case for a couple of thousand years after the initial herds were formed.

Then, imagine a bucolic scene in a Neolithic meadow one day 7,500 years ago, where a proto-cowboy was looking after the cattle, and watching a cow suckle its calf, when there was a sudden 'Eureka' (or whatever a Neolithic cowboy might appropriately say in that situation) moment. Humans at the time would, of course, have been familiar with breast-feeding their infants. Putting two and two together, so to speak, and realising that they could also consume the milk of herd animals, however, was another step-change in the development of human civilisation. Milking or 'dairying' would have provided energy and nutrients without the need to slaughter precious livestock and simply using the animals for meat. For example, the amount of milk produced by a Neolithic cow has been estimated at between 400 and 600 litres for each weaning period, with cows typically producing one calf per year. Even when taking into account the milk necessary to feed the growing calves, some 150–250 litres would be left for humans to drink.[5] This is almost equivalent to the amount of calories available from the meat of a whole cow. This would have been per animal, per year, and long before selective breeding began to dramatically increase milk yield. Today, a modern Holstein Friesian dairy cow will produce an average of 10,000 litres of milk per year! Keeping in mind that even with farming and agriculture, humans never had enough to eat (in fact it is probably only thirty to forty years ago that we had 'too much' to eat), this new stream of calories would have been immensely beneficial to nascent pastoralists.

THE CHEESEMAKERS

Nutritious though it was, the major problem with milk was that it only lasted for a couple of days before turning sour; less than a day in hotter climes. It was only with the advent of milk pasteurisation in the early 1900s that the (refrigerated) shelf-life of milk was extended to the two weeks we expect today. So for the vast majority of human existence, milk was impossible to store for any length of time or transport over any significant distance.

However, let's return to the proto-cowboy sitting in that meadow of Neolithic cattle some 7,500 years ago. Imagine one day, as he was enjoying a (clay pottery) beaker of milk fresh from the cow, he might have, in a fit of generosity, decided to bring some back to share his enjoyment with the rest of his village. He transferred the milk into containers made from cows' (or sheep's) stomachs, which were waterproof and pretty much unbreakable, brought them back home, and everyone got to enjoy a nice calcium- and vitamin-D-rich nutritious beverage. But one stomach full of milk was forgotten about, and it sat out in the open overnight. The next day, our cowboy noticed the rogue pouch, and opened it up to see if the contents were still drinkable. Instead of milk, what he found was a white solid sitting in a clear liquid. When he warily sampled it, he found that it tasted a bit sour, and because he didn't immediately keel over from food poisoning, nor experience any other negative gastrointestinal effects, he concluded that it was otherwise edible. What he had serendipitously discovered were curds (the solid) and whey (the liquid), the first step in the cheesemaking process. A number of variations of this myth exist, set in central Asia or the fertile crescent or central Europe, and sometimes replacing the cow with a sheep or a goat.

The development of the process to turn milk into cheese ranks, with yeast-leavened bread and the fermentation of alcoholic beverages, as one of our most important agricultural technological achievements. It enabled us to convert a nutritious drink that had to be consumed immediately, lest it spoiled, to a product that would last; with many cheeses, if stored correctly, staying unspoilt for years. In addition, because cheese is a solid, it is more nutritionally dense than milk and far easier to transport, which meant that it could be used as a portable source of food.

Milk is, of course, mostly water. The principle of cheesemaking, in essence, is to take the fat and protein in milk and turn it into a solid by removing much of the water, while preserving and flavouring it through acidification and the addition of salt. As a general rule, the more water that is removed, the drier and harder the cheese, and the longer it will last. Parmigiano-Reggiano or Parmesan, for example, is one of the hardest cheeses available. It takes two years to make and mature, and has a shelf life of easily another year. As an aside, I really don't know why the blocks of Parmesan you buy from a supermarket come with a 'best by' date at all. It has taken more than two years to get to your fridge, and it will suddenly go off in two weeks? Please. If kept in the fridge, the Parmesan might get drier and harder, but it will last for years, with no loss in nutritional value. This from a starting material that lasts no more than a couple of days.

LITTLE MISS MUFFET

The first step in the cheesemaking process is separating the milk into curds and whey. Every time I say curds and whey, like a Rorschach test, this nursery rhyme immediately springs to mind:

> *Little Miss Muffet*
> *Sat on a tuffet,*
> *Eating her curds and whey;*
> *Along came a spider*
> *Who sat down beside her*
> *And frightened Miss Muffet away.*

As with most kids, I recited this rhyme without knowing its meaning. In fact, to this day, I still have no idea who Miss Muffet was, why she was sitting on a tuffet, or what, for that matter, a tuffet is; but I do know about curds and whey. These are made when milk is gently heated, and then rennet and bacterial 'starter cultures' added. Rennet is a complex of proteins that are produced in the stomachs of ruminants such as cows or sheep. What it does is to coagulate casein, the primary type of protein present in milk, to form the curd. The bacterial culture ferments the lactose in milk into lactic acid. This is an accelerated process of what happens at home, when bacteria inevitably gets into the milk, producing lactic acid and making it taste sour; hence the 'souring' of milk. Tweaking the amount of rennet used influences the speed of the curd formation, and varying the mix of bacteria in the 'starter culture' changes the speed of acidification and thus the final level of acidity reached. Mix in the amount and length of salting, and how much whey is removed through pressing, these are then all factors that will determine what style of cheese will be created before it is matured. The climate would also have influenced the types of cheese produced, with cooler temperatures requiring less salt for preservation, for instance. The earliest cheeses were likely to have been quite sour and salty, probably similar in taste and texture to cottage cheese or feta.

Depending on the levels of salt and acidity, some cheeses then became a suitable medium for certain microbes and moulds, adding another layer of complexity and distinctive flavours. This would, once again, have occurred by chance, and then been honed by trial and error. I have often wondered about the first *fromagère* (French for cheesemaker, oh la la) happening upon a cheese that had gone 'blue' with mould, who was then brave (is crazy a better adjective?) enough to try it! I am grateful to that pioneering reckless cheesemaker, though, because a fine piece of blue Stilton on a cracker, accompanied by a dollop of quince jelly, and maybe served with some port wine, is a rare pleasure indeed (OMG, I think I have spent too long in Cambridge).

So the story of the Neolithic cowboy and all its variations is not as apocryphal as you would think. Clearly, I have taken dramatic licence in its telling and the exact scenario can only be left to our imagination. However, animal skins and inflated internal organs are known to have provided storage vessels for a range of foodstuffs. The residual rennet left in a cow's stomach, coupled with the milk within being heated by the sun, would have been enough to trigger the production of curds and whey, and it is probable that cheese was discovered by accident in this fashion. But it need not have been the only way.

In fact, cheesemaking was probably developed independently, multiple times, simply because of how easily and often milk does go off. The acidification of milk by bacterial fermentation would, without the addition of any rennet, also have curdled milk. We have all experienced this with the pint of milk we'd forgotten about in the fridge before going on vacation that by the time we get back has turned into a gelatinous solid. This curdled milk could have been preserved by pressing (to remove water) and salting. Then when Neolithic pastoralists realised that an animal stomach gave more solid and better-textured curds, and therefore better cheese, it may have led to the deliberate addition of rennet.

Both milk and cheese have broadly the same nutritional make-up, albeit concentrated into a far smaller volume in the latter, with the exception of the levels of lactose. An unintended consequence of converting milk into cheese is that much of the lactose ends up being removed. Some of it is, of course, fermented into lactic acid; but the vast majority of lactose stays in solution in the whey, during the process where the fat and protein coagulates into curds. So, for instance, while lactose levels in milk are around 5 per cent, it is only 0.07 per cent of Cheddar or Parmesan. That is a greater than 70-fold reduction of lactose. As a general rule, the softer the cheese, the more lactose it contains. Ricotta, for example, can contain up to 3 per cent lactose. Whey, as a comparison, is 50–75 per cent lactose! As a result, many cheeses are actually far more easily digested than milk, even amongst lactose-intolerant folks.

Cheese, this renewable, portable and nutritionally dense new source of food, ended up playing an important role in helping nascent pastoral communities thrive and grow, and in the case of Europe, expand across an entire continent.

YOGURT

Another method of extending the life of milk was to turn it into yogurt. Frank Kosikowski and Vikram Mistry in their 1997 tome *Cheese and Fermented Milk Foods, Volume 1*, suggest that yogurt was probably discovered by the ancient Mesopotamians about 7,000 years ago. It was most likely discovered in a similar way to cheese; that is, by accident, when bacteria within an old goat (or sheep) stomach began to ferment the milk it contained. The main difference with yogurt is that the milk solids are not separated out, and thus it remains in liquid form. In order to produce yogurt, milk is first heated, to denature the protein so that it does not form curds. The temperature at which this first heating step takes place and the protein content of the starting milk influences the thickness and creaminess of the yogurt. The higher the denaturing temperature and amount of protein, the thicker and creamier the final yogurt. After the protein is denatured, a bacterial culture is then mixed in, and fermentation allowed to occur for up to twelve hours. Once again, our Neolithic pastoralists would have had to work the process out over time and through trial and error.

Yogurt is produced using a culture of *Lactobacillus delbrueckii* and *Streptococcus thermophilus* bacteria, and these bacteria for the most part remain alive in the final product. It is, in effect, a live bacterial culture; the original 'pro-biotic'. These bacteria are clearly not harmful to us; in fact, they are of benefit to our gut health. Yogurt is one of the original 'health foods', thought to have curative properties. Whether or not this is true is debatable, with a lack of enough clinical trial data to conclude that consuming yogurt lowers risk of diseases or improves health. But what is clear is that it is highly nutritious. In addition, the presence of the live bacteria continuing to break down the lactose makes yogurt, like cheese, easier to digest.

MILK IS A SAFE DRINKING SOURCE

The reason that milk spoils so quickly is because it is such a rich medium for bacteria to grow. As I mentioned in Chapter 4, the US Center for Disease Control (CDC) says that improperly handled unpasteurised or 'raw' milk is responsible for nearly three times more hospitalisations than any other food-borne disease source, making it one of the world's most dangerous food products. Now I am certainly not advocating that everyone runs out and starts drinking raw milk. That being said, if there was nothing else at all to drink, such as in the desert and other arid regions, then fresh milk immediately out of a cow/sheep/goat/camel (camel milk, while not available at your local supermarket or espresso bar, is understandably very popular in desert areas) was an important drinking source. Considering the symptoms of lactose intolerance, which include water loss from diarrhoea, individuals who had acquired the genetic adaptation of 'lactase persistence' and could therefore drink and metabolise milk would have had a very strong selective advantage in areas where herding of ruminants occurred.

LACTASE PERSISTENCE

The Neolithic *Linearbandkeramik* (German for 'linear pottery') people, so called for the decorative technique of lines used on the pottery associated with this culture, arrived in Europe 7,500 years ago. Archaeological evidence revealed not only the type of pottery used by this group of people, but also that they reared cattle. In fact, it was likely that the *Linearbandkeramik* introduced both the rearing of cattle and dairying to Europe.[6] How do we know this? Well, DNA evidence shows that the emergence of the genetic change resulting in lactase persistence, enabling Europeans to drink milk as adults and not feel ill, had its origins with these people with a penchant for line-decorated pottery.

As I mentioned at the outset of this chapter, all humans (all mammals) are able to drink milk when they are very young. They do this by expressing lactase within the small intestine, which breaks down the lactose present in milk into glucose and galactose that are then absorbed by the body. What happens in most mammals as they stop breast-feeding and begin to eat solid food, is that lactase levels fall away. This occurs when another protein comes along and binds to a segment of DNA next to the *Lactase* gene, and in doing so, turns the gene off, stopping the production of lactase. Around 7,500 years ago, someone amongst the linear pottery pastoralists developed a mutation within this segment of DNA, which scientists called the -13,910*T allele (catchy!).[7]

In Chapter 1, I introduced the concept that mutations within our DNA happen randomly and at a low background level all of the time. Most of the time, these changes have no measurable effect. Rarely, a mutation ends up altering the function of a gene. If a resulting change is not desirable in a certain environment, then it is 'selected against' and not passed on. If, however, the functional change increases your chances of survival, then it is 'selected for' and that mutation is then passed on and integrates itself into the population. This was one of those rare situations where a mutation did alter the function of a gene in a positive fashion. What the -13,910*T allele did was to prevent the protein that turned off the *Lactase* gene from binding to the adjacent segment of DNA. As a result, this person's *Lactase* gene was never turned off, leading to the continued expression of lactase in his or her small intestine in adulthood, and the ability of the lucky person, perhaps our Neolithic cowboy, to drink milk throughout their life. It is difficult to know exactly when this mutation occurred, but we do know that it was brought into Europe by the *Linearbandkeramik*. The ability to consume dairy products was so advantageous that the

-13,910*T allele spread throughout all of Europe. Today, the frequency of lactase persistence is between 15 per cent and 54 per cent in Eastern and Southern Europe, 62 per cent and 86 per cent in Central and Western Europe, and up to more than 90 per cent of the populations in the British Isles and Scandinavia.[8] Nearly all of these Europeans with lactase persistence carry the -13,910*T allele. Hooray for the *Linearbandkeramik*!

Given that the *Linearbandkeramik* introduced dairying to Europe, it is perhaps not surprising that the earliest evidence for cheesemaking can also be traced back to them. Archaeologists had recovered fragments of linear pottery pierced with small holes around 2–3 millimetres in diameter from a 7,500-year-old *Linearbandkeramik* site. When organic material left behind on the pottery fragments was chemically analysed, it was unequivocally dairy in origin. However, the critical finding was the high-fat content in the residue, which was consistent with it coming from curds, as opposed to the lower fat content found in milk.[9] During the cheesemaking process, the next step after the coagulation of milk is the separation of the liquid whey away from the solid curds. Today, this straining or pressing process is commonly achieved using a 'cheesecloth' or, depending on the type of cheese being made, plastic or metal sieves. These pierced linear pottery fragments had come from a clay sieve, a Neolithic 'cheese-strainer', and represented the earliest evidence of cheesemaking.

It is interesting how early cheesemaking began, right at the dawn of dairying, and at the time when the -13,910*T allele began to undergo selection and to spread. Since milk spoilt so easily, there was certainly plenty of opportunity for our Neolithic cowboy to accidentally discover curds. Also, because removing the whey from the curds strips out much of the lactose, cheese actually ends up having quite a low lactose content, making it far easier to digest than milk. This would have been important early on, before the

-13,910*T allele became as widespread as today, for early pastoralists to enjoy the nutritional benefits of milk, without having to necessarily drink milk.

Just a bit of nerdy detail for those (like me) who care; scientists modelling the spread of the -13,910*T allele do not think it happened at an even rate.[10] Evidence suggests that during times of plenty, when there would have been lots of grain available and the newly discovered 'lactose-lite' cheese to eat, the positive selection for lactase persistence may have been relatively weak. However, under certain episodic circumstances, such as drought, epidemic or famine, or even in between harvesting seasons, milk would have represented an alternative food resource, and then those who were lactase persistent would have had a selective advantage. Multiple episodic selection events over more than a thousand years led to the -13,910*T allele being spread throughout Europe.

CONVERGENT PERSISTENCE

So powerful was the selection pressure in herding societies to be able to consume milk and its related products that the trait of lactase persistence actually emerged independently at least three times; in Europeans, as we've discussed, and in two geographically distinct populations in Eastern Africa and the Fulani in central Africa.[11] The incredible thing is that although the adaptation in the three cases involved different genetic changes, they all influenced the *Lactase* gene in the same fashion. For instance, one of the East African variants is called the -14,010*C allele, which is physically very close to the -13,910*T allele, and also prevents the protein that turns off the *Lactase* gene from binding that segment of DNA. Thus, lactase levels remain high in East Africans, even in adulthood. This is a classic example of what is known as 'convergent evolution,' where two completely distinct populations have independently developed exactly the same strategy, albeit with different genetic changes, to be able to digest lactose in adulthood.

SIXTY-FIVE PER CENT OF ADULT HUMANS ARE LACTOSE INTOLERANT

But, and it is a very important but, only 35 per cent of adult humans today are lactase persistent. The other 65 per cent of adults, most of the world outside of Europe and North America essentially, are lactose intolerant. Given all of the many advantages of consuming dairy products, how have most other peoples around the world continued to thrive without this ability, even till today, to digest lactose as adults? While the answer to this question is clearly going to be different depending on which culture or people we are talking about, there is a universal truth; in order for a culture to not only survive, but to thrive, there had to be enough calories, particularly from protein, available to the population. I am ethnically Chinese and although my fluency in the language (Mandarin 普通话, the common tongue, and Teo Chew 潮州, my dialect) is more than a little suspect (much to the disappointment of my mother), I am deeply familiar with Chinese food culture, both from the perspective of cooking and eating (much to my mother's relief), and will use it here as a case study.

1. *The chicken came first*

Cattle rearing was never a 'thing' in China, or in most of East Asia for that matter. Certainly the climate in much of East Asia would not have precluded the herding of cattle. So, in lieu of viable milking herds, what were the alternative sources of easily renewable protein? For one thing, the Chinese were the first to domesticate the chicken (*Gallus domesticus*) from the red jungle fowl (*Gallus gallus*).[12] Researchers have found the earliest evidence for chicken domestication in an area around the Yellow River in northern China, with DNA obtained from the 10,500-year-old fossilised bones confirming that they belonged to the same lineage as modern domestic chickens.[13] That matches the date of domestication of the first mammals (sheep and goats) in central Asia. Thus, in China, from the very beginning of the agricultural revolution, chickens, as opposed to mammals, were 'first out of the block' and formed an important early farmed source of protein for the Neolithic Chinese. The protein came not only from the meat, but obviously also from eggs, which, like cheese, were a rich, portable and renewable food source. In fact, for most of the year, except from when they were moulting, hens lay an egg nearly every day. Chickens were also far smaller, had a shorter lifespan and therefore a faster breeding cycle, as compared to large mammalian species, which made their rearing far easier. It also meant that some could be bred exclusively for the purpose of meat and others for egg laying.

2. We don't drink pig milk

Then, a couple of thousand years after the chicken (or was it the egg?), the Chinese domesticated the pig (*Sus scrofa*) from the wild boar. For the Chinese this was the first large mammal 'tamed' for the purposes of meat. The pig was actually domesticated independently twice. Once in Anatolia, what is now Turkey, around 9,000–10,000 years ago, and then again in China, nearly 9,000 years ago, at the Neolithic Jiahu site.[14] Jiahu is in east central China between the Yellow and Yangtze Rivers. It is interesting to note that while the pig is clearly a mammal, we certainly do not drink pig milk. There appear to be multiple reasons for this. A cow has a temperament that is conducive to milking: they stand placidly and lactate, allowing easy access for the human and calf to the udder. Goats can be a little more uncooperative but easily manoeuvred due to their small size. Milking a pig is a much more difficult undertaking; omnivores feed their young lying down, making human access to the multiple teats more difficult, so there is a mechanical restriction. Persuading a lactating 250-pound pig with a protective instinct for her litter to part with her milk is not straightforward and frankly rather dangerous. I suspect the key reason, however, why pigs have not been utilised for milk production, may be the cost benefit of taking milk from a pig versus allowing the pig to utilise its food to accumulate meat and fat and produce two litters of piglets a year. Cows have the added advantage that they can still become pregnant despite lactating, whereas pigs will only become receptive to mating once they have weaned their litter. As a consequence, humans only drink the milk of humans (of course, but, aside for infants, ick!) and ruminants, and not of omnivores or carnivores (I now have an image in my head of someone trying to milk a tiger, with disastrous consequences).

As a result of these domestication events, for much of history, chickens and pigs formed the bulk of the meat consumed in East Asia. Ruminants were simply not reared on any significant scale, and hence dairying never took root. There was therefore no reason, no pressure, for the lactase persistence trait to be selected for.

3. *Tofu glorious tofu*
Crucially, one of the key crops domesticated by the Chinese, in addition to rice of course, was the soybean. Soybeans are legumes, which are notable in that most of them have symbiotic nitrogen-fixing bacteria in structures in their roots called nodules. Nitrogen is essential for plant growth and development; well, for all life actually, but all non-plant life get their fill of nitrogen by eating plants or animals. The problem is that plants can't utilise the nitrogen that forms 78 per cent of air. Most plants instead depend upon combined or fixed forms of nitrogen, such as ammonia and nitrate. This will come from animal waste, decomposition of

dead plants and animals, or fertilisers. Some plants, however, like legumes, can 'fix' atmospheric nitrogen into usable form through symbiosis with the bacteria in their root nodules, for themselves initially, but then becoming available to neighbouring or subsequent plants over time, through root dieback or fallen leaves and other material. Soybeans are one of these nitrogen-fixing plants, and for that reason, they play a key role in crop rotation, helping to 'fix' nitrogen into the soil, for other crops to benefit from. While the earliest historical record for soybean use comes from the Shang dynasty, sometime between 1700–1100 BC, archaeological evidence dates its domestication in China to between 6,000 and 9,000 years ago, although where exactly is still unclear.[15] Certainly the charred plant remains of wild soybean have been recovered from Neolithic Jiahu, the same place where the remains of the first domesticated pigs were found.

The first key point about the soybean is its versatility. It is the source ingredient for tofu, soymilk, fermented soybeans (including the yellow and black beans from the respective eponymous sauces), and a dizzying array of different soy sauces; from the thick and sweet Kecap manis (the crude oil of the soy sauce world) and dark soy sauce, to the light salty soy sauce in ubiquitous use today. The second important point about the soybean is its very high protein content, even in its derived products. For example, tofu and soy sauce both contain 8 per cent protein. Tofu I'm not at all surprised about. But 8 per cent protein in soy sauce? The stuff you flavour your stir-fries with and dip your sushi into? I was certainly very surprised when I found out. This is compared to the 3.3 per cent protein found in soymilk, which is almost identical to the amount of protein found in milk. Thus, because it is used in so many ways and in pretty much every single meal, the soybean has, and continues to be, a key protein source in East Asia.

So where do the Chinese get their protein from in lieu of milk? Chickens, pigs and tofu. As they never had the need to drink milk, there was no selection pressure for them to become lactase persistent.

NO MORE CAPPUCCINOS

I have, until very recently, always thought that lactose-intolerant folk were going to be all very much like my dad, in that he could not touch a drop of milk or a crumb of cheese. Mom was very different. When the opportunity presented itself, she could and would enjoy a slice of pizza or a piece of cheesecake or some yogurt. As you might have gathered from my culinary exploits in my early months in San Francisco, I take after my mother. With my geneticist head on, I just assumed that my dad did not carry any of the genetic variations associated with lactase persistence, such as the 13,910*T allele. Whereas my mom probably carried one of these alleles, which I then inherited, explaining why both of us were lactose persistent. At least that was what I thought.

I was contacted recently by a health journalist of a major UK tabloid newspaper, asking if I would review one of these new-fangled genetic tests, which claimed to be able to make predictions about your health, disease, physical traits and capabilities. They offered to pay for me to get genetically tested by this particular company, and then to give my opinion of the results and their interpretation. From the perspective of intellectual curiosity, it seemed too good an opportunity to miss, so I agreed. I will give a full review of the test in Chapter 12, but suffice to say, I entered into this enterprise deeply sceptical. When the results came back, I quickly swiped through to get a general feel of the data provided and how it was being interpreted. So for instance, based on my genetic information, I was likely not to be coeliac (correct) and I had a heterozygous genetic variant at my *Alcohol Dehydrogenase*

1C gene,[16] which meant that while I could metabolise alcohol, I couldn't drink as much as many of my white Caucasian friends (correct). But then I got to the section about lactase persistence, and did a double take. In big bold letters, it said:

'Your result means that you, like the majority of the world population, do not possess the variant that causes lactase persistence therefore it is strongly recommended that you avoid/reduce lactose.'

Strongly recommended that I avoid or reduce lactose. Really? I was certain that the genetic result, which was empirical, would be correct, but yet I was eating dairy on a near daily basis. I called up my mom and asked her if she thought she was lactose intolerant. She said of course! She couldn't drink milk, but could eat cheese and yogurt, as long as she didn't overdo it.

'Aren't you the same?' she asked.

I'm sure no one will believe me, but I had never given it any thought before. Ridiculous, I know.

My favourite morning poison used to be a cappuccino; one of those from an espresso bar that comes in a pint-sized insulated paper cup, with three shots of strong coffee, quite a bit of milk, and topped off with a frothy lid sprinkled with cocoa powder. I loved it. I had never really been a breakfast cereal or porridge oats person (I now know why), so the only milk I would have had on a daily basis would have been in my coffee. I was then curious to experiment and see what would happen if I shifted to black Americanos in the morning instead. After a couple of mornings of black coffee, certain *ahem* symptoms went away. I then performed the 'crossover', where I went back on to cappuccinos for just a couple of days; lo and behold, the symptoms returned. I do appreciate that this was not an experiment as such; for one thing it was not 'blinded' and since it only had one participant, i.e. me, it could really only be considered anecdotal. However, in my defence, my 'self-diagnosis' was backed up by a genetic test.

My name is Giles Yeo, and apparently, in my mid-forties, I have just learnt that I am lactose intolerant.

SOME PEOPLE ARE MORE INTOLERANT THAN OTHERS

I now know that not all people with lactase deficiency and lactose malabsorption have digestive symptoms. My nutritionist colleagues tell me that adults and adolescents with lactose intolerance can eat or drink up to 12 grams of lactose in one sitting, equating to the amount of lactose in 1 cup of milk, without symptoms or with only minor symptoms. But as you can see from my family, lactose-intolerant individuals clearly vary in the amount of lactose they can tolerate. My dad sits on one end of the spectrum, suffering from severe symptoms even after a small amount of dairy; I mean, I don't think he would be able to watch a Pizza Hut commercial without going into gastrointestinal distress. I, on the other hand, can and do eat yogurt and cheese quite happily without having digestive symptoms, even while not being able to drink much milk.

Given my recent journey of self-discovery into lactose intolerance, I have suddenly acquired an interest in the lactose content of various dairy products. As discussed in this chapter, many cheeses have a near negligible lactose content, and while yogurt does contain nearly as much as milk, it is digested more efficiently than other dairy sources due to the live bacteria present, which facilitates lactose digestion. Therefore, fermented dairy products, such as yoghurt, soured cream, crème fraîche and many cheeses, are typically well tolerated by many lactose-intolerant individuals. As a general rule of thumb, the higher the fat content, the lower the lactose content. So for example, soured cream is 10 per cent fat and contains 3.6 per cent lactose, while crème fraîche is 30 per cent fat and contains 2.4 per cent lactose. As for cheese, the harder it is, the less lactose it will contain.

WHY BE DAIRY FREE? LET ME COUNT THE WAYS . . .

Aside from biological constraints, people do choose to be dairy-free for other reasons, which might be ethical, environmental or health-related; I will address these issues in detail in the next chapter. There are also cultural or religious reasons to avoid dairy products. I was speaking at the Israeli Society for Neuroscience Annual meeting in 2017, which was being held at the Dead Sea resort of Eilat. All of the speakers and most of the delegates stayed in the fancy and very large hotel that was attached to the convention centre. In the evening, everyone ate at the enormous hotel restaurant, which provided a dinner buffet that would rival in size anything you could find in Las Vegas, and the food that was served was excellent. It was also unusual, compared to the buffets you would find in Vegas, or for that matter compared to most of the restaurants you would find in the UK or the US, in the amount of vegetables that was served. Raw in salads, roasted in olive oil and herbs, pickled, stir-fried, the list went on. I would have said more than 50 per cent of the length of the buffet provided vegetables of some description. This was even true for breakfast! Vegetables for breakfast! The restaurant had a Kashrut Certificate, meaning that all the food that was served was Kosher, thus obeying all of the Jewish food laws. Out of curiosity, I asked my hosts what proportion of Israeli Jews would observe the kosher rules. They told me that around 40 per cent of the population observed kosher laws to some degree; however, a hotel of the size we were in, or of any size really, could not afford to alienate any potential business, so it was simpler to just be entirely kosher. One of these food laws forbids the mixture of meat and milk, and is thought to be based on two verses in the Book of Exodus, which forbade 'boiling a (kid) goat in its mother's milk'.[17] While I was previously familiar with this rule, I had not realised the details with regards to timing. So after eating meat, you have to wait at least six hours before consuming any dairy, presumably just in case you have any meat stuck in your teeth. In the reciprocal situation, you have to wait anywhere between thirty minutes to three hours after consuming dairy (it depends who you ask and how strictly they adhere to the laws), before you can eat meat. Rather than deal with the complexity of who can eat what, when and where, dinner was an entirely dairy-free affair. Not a single bit of cheese or cream in any of the food, not even the desserts! It was all very, very good; if no one had informed me, I would have been none the wiser. This is apparently true of many eating establishments in Israel.

As I've mentioned, I spent a significant period of my childhood in Singapore where, in the 1980s, fresh milk was almost non-existent. Singapore is a tiny place, a diamond-shaped island roughly 26 miles from east to west and 15 miles from north to south. Back then, there were just over two million people crammed on to the island; today, the population is over four million. It was so small that pretty much everything, even including water, had to be brought in. There was certainly no grazing area for any livestock, and so very little fresh milk. Powdered skimmed milk was available, and I used to be made to drink a small cup every morning by my mum, because it was good for my bones she said. I don't remember ever enjoying the experience because it was just so awful ... up there with cod-liver oil (yuck ... who ever thought fishy-flavoured mayonnaise was a good idea?). Perhaps the technology required to manufacture powdered milk without the terrible taste has improved in the 21st century, but due to my conditioned taste aversion to it, I haven't tried any since I was eight years old! In truth, the real reason that there was no fresh milk in Singapore was because 75 per cent of the population were Chinese, and therefore the vast majority were lactose intolerant. Thus, everyone drank soy milk. But we drank it as it was, we never put it in tea or coffee or our cereal. Today, however, because it is perceived by some to be a healthier option than cow's milk, it is widely available in all major supermarkets and in most coffee shops all over the world as a milk replacement.

BLESSED ARE THE CHEESEMAKERS

Is consuming dairy bad for you *per se*? Having scoured the literature, the consensus appears to be that consumption of dairy does not lead to increases in heart disease and all-cause mortality (the cheerfully euphemistic scientific term for death). It doesn't appear to improve your health, but it is certainly not bad for you.[18] There are layers of nuance in the data, though. So, for example, dairy consumption in children and adolescents is actually associated with reduced body fat and increased muscle mass.[19] Thus, un-surprisingly, milk is important earlier on in life, to ensure proper growth. Another study, this time in adults, suggested that whole milk consumption may be directly associated with cancer mortal-ity, while non-fat milk consumption was actually protective.[20] This is only one study, though, and will need replication by someone else before it can be considered reliable. But if you take it at face value, then it argues that the fat in the milk is the problem, rather than the milk itself.

But here is the reality. As with ALL mammals, we have evolved to drink milk as infants and in childhood. If, like my dad and (now I know) me, you are lactose intolerant as an adult, then choosing the decaf soy latte or sticking to black Americanos is probably wise. However, lactose is a sugar, and is the same no matter which type of milk it is found in. So, if you have the genetic adaptation allowing you to be lactase persistent as an adult, then milk, whether from humans (ick), cows, sheep, goats or camels, is not going to be bad for you. Unless of course you have too much of it, which can lead to obesity. That, however, is not a problem with dairy, but a problem with the number of calories. But there is no denying that the ability to digest cow (and goat and sheep and camel) milk and its products gave some humans the edge in the survival stakes and helped them thrive in early agricultural societies.

PART 3

Let food be thy medicine

'Let food be thy medicine and medicine be thy food.'
'If we could give every individual the right amount
    of nourishment and exercise, not too little and not
    too much, we would have found the safest way to
    health.'
'Everything in excess is opposed to nature.'
'All disease begins in the gut.'

— Hippocrates

CHAPTER 7

I am 'plant-based', NOT a vegan

'Food Matters Live' is held at ExCeL London in November every year. It is what is known as a 'cross-sector' event, bringing together the food and drink industry, policy makers as well as scientists, dieticians and other professionals working in nutrition and health, combining a mixture of talks, panel discussions and demonstrations within a large exhibition floor. A big food 'love-in' of sorts. I was invited in 2017 to take part in a discussion panel on the main stage, entitled 'From psychology to marketing: what influences healthier food choices?'

ExCeL is an enormous exhibition venue located on the north quay of the Royal Victoria Dock in London Docklands, between Canary Wharf and London City Airport. As a non-Londoner, my entire geographical understanding of the capital is from the perspective of the Tube system (or subway or metro, depending on where you hail from). I would know, for example, that two locations were six stops and one line-change apart on the Tube, maybe a 20-minute journey; but have no idea that on the surface world, they were actually less than half a mile apart, a 10-minute jaunt at the very most. So one of the scariest things you can do (for me anyway) is to actually leave the Tube system and have to negotiate your way through alternative transport systems such as the London Overground commuter rail or even flag down a bus (heaven forbid). To get to London ExCeL, I needed to leave the Tube at Bank station, and get on to the Docklands Light Rail (DLR). I alighted at Prince Regent Station and made my way into ExCeL through its East entrance.

It was my first time attending, and with the caveat that I was only there for one day, most of the speakers were well known and respected in their fields, and their presentations appeared to be evidence-based. The exhibitors were, however, shall we say, a mixed bag. There was an education and research section, where the major nutritional institutes as well as funding and professional bodies all had stands, although they were by far and away in the minority. As for the rest of the exhibitors, half of them were trying to get you to eat more of their various wares, and the other half were trying to get you to eat less of one thing or another. Some things made sense, with a large low-sugar and sugar-replacement section, for instance. Others were definitely on the faddy end of the dietary spectrum. There was a glut of gluten-free products, which I'm certain were not actually being marketed towards those with coeliac disease. There definitely was pH 9 water available in all of its alkaline goodness (we'll return to this in Chapter 9). Lots of stuff with turmeric, for its anti-cancerous properties apparently; and then there was 'protein cheese' . . . I know, there is nothing more to say.

During my panel discussions, there were four other people on the stage with me: Dr Lauren McGale, a food psychologist from Liverpool University; the food historian Dr Annie Gray; the chef Anthony Warner, whose alter-ego is the acerbic writer and food blogger 'The Angry Chef'; and the BBC Radio 4 presenter Timandra Harkness, who was tasked with moderating the discussion amongst the panel, and also fielding questions from the floor. We all work on food choice, but from very different perspectives, so I found it very interesting and enlightening; all in all, it was an enjoyable and lively session.

As we were stepping off stage, there was a rush of people coming up to speak to each of the panellists. A number of the audience recognised me from my *Clean Eating* documentary that had screened earlier in the year; this was a food event after all. So there were people seeking advice about diets, requests for selfies, and also a number of science-related questions. While this was all happening, a young man rushed into the middle of the scrum. He said how interesting he found my work and asked whether I would be willing to answer a few questions about the genetics of obesity for his podcast? Given that I was already giving a couple of other interviews, including one for the Food Matters Live organisers, it seemed an entirely appropriate and innocent enough request, so I agreed.

After I had fulfilled my other interview commitments and things had quietened down, I sat down with the young man at the designated 'media area', where he had a colleague operating a camcorder on a tripod. The interview began, as they very often do, with questions about the role of genes in obesity, the role of the environment and how the brain is involved. A few minutes in, the questions shifted to my motivation for making the *Clean Eating* documentary. Up until then, the interview had been good-natured and moving along exactly as I had expected. Then everything changed abruptly. There came a quick series of questions, each with an increasing level of aggressiveness:

'Tell us about the pushback you've been getting online to your film?'

'Isn't it true that you are paid by a drug company and have no interest to see diets work?'

'Are you not a self-confessed unchangeable carnivore who refuses to believe in the plant-based diet?'

The penny dropped in the middle of the second question, and by the third, I realised, with a sinking feeling, that I had been ambushed.

QUEEN ELLA

The BBC's Horizon documentary about the 'clean eating' phenomenon was 'green lit' in the early summer of 2016. When production began, we knew that we wanted to try and land an interview with one of the key drivers of the movement. We reached out to a number of the big beasts, including Natasha Corrett of Honestly Healthy and the Hemsley sisters, Jasmine and Melissa, more in hope than in expectation. The director and producer of the documentary was Tristan Quinn, and his ethos was to be as open with the reasons for our investigation as was reasonably possible, and also with the fact that I would be approaching the interview from a position of scepticism. I therefore did not think that their public relations teams would let us anywhere near them, and I was not surprised when Natasha declined our invitation and we got no response from the Hemsleys. There was, however, no one bigger than Ella Mills (*née* Woodward), otherwise known as Deliciously Ella. Her début cookbook was the fastest selling, ever, in the UK, and she had more than a million followers on Instagram. Her recipes, at least in her first two books *Deliciously Ella* and (just in case you couldn't get enough of Ella) *Deliciously Ella Every Day*, are vegan (this appears to be a bad word in the plant-based community; more on this later), as well as refined sugar-, gluten- and dairy-free. Ella's team *did* respond to our request. This led to a couple of exploratory meetings, including one where Ella and I met in person, so she could sniff me out. We let her know that while we would supply the broad topics for discussion beforehand, there would be no questions barred, but she could choose whether or not to respond. Much to my surprise, in spite of the conditions, she agreed to be interviewed by me on camera.

The BBC had rented a large studio apartment for the purposes of filming a number of scenes. It occupied the second floor of a trendy converted warehouse, and was spaciously open plan, with high ceilings, skylights, as well as exposed piping and brickwork. The centrepiece of the studio was a large fabulous kitchen (I will admit kitchen envy), and the plan was for me to cook for Ella (eek!), while conducting the interview. Every so often, you find yourself questioning your life choices . . . this was one of those moments.

I am a fair home cook, so I do know my way around a kitchen. The problem was, I don't typically cook many vegan dishes; I maybe have four or five in my repertoire. I could hardly have produced a steak for Ella, because that would simply have been rude. Plus, there was the small matter of the interview and the whole event being captured on camera for primetime TV! This was a valuable once-in-a-lifetime opportunity and I needed to put a strategy in place to make sure I didn't screw it up. In the end, I decided to cook one of Ella's own recipes, because it would act as a natural talking point through which to structure the questions (I don't like to use notes, preferring to have organic cues to nudge me to the next point, which allows for a more conversational tone). I chose her spiced sweet potato stew, because it seemed simple enough for me to prepare whilst conducting an interview; lots of peeling of sweet potatoes and simmering and stirring, and therefore lots of time and space to cogitate on plant-based thoughts.

It was a cold autumn day in November when we shot the interview. Thankfully, the rain stayed away, so when Ella eventually made it up the stairs and into the apartment, after filming all of the necessary shots to 'establish' her coming to visit me (I'm told you just cannot have someone apparently teleport into a scene), she still looked her radiant self. Ella is ridiculously good-looking; you can't help a sharp intake of breath and a sneaky second glance, resulting in a stiff elbow in the ribs from the missus, type of good-looking. Once Ella stepped into the apartment, the cameras began rolling, and the whole cooking scene and interview was filmed as 'actuality'; meaning it was done in one long take, with the camera just following us around. After a bit, you kinda forgot the camera was there, which was the whole point of the exercise, I guess.

'Have you always been a plant lover?'

'No, God – oh my God, no. I was actually the worst – I was the least vegetarian person you would have ever met in your life – ten years ago. Hated vegetables. Hated fruit.'

Eleanor 'Ella' Laura Davan Woodward is the daughter of Shaun Woodward, a British politician and Camilla, heiress to the Sainsbury's supermarket empire. Thus, she had good genes and was undoubtedly born into substance. In her late teens, while still an undergraduate, she did a stint as a model. But suddenly at nineteen years old, she came down with a rare condition called Postural Orthostatic Tachycardia Syndrome or POTS. POTS is a condition in which standing up quickly from a lying down position results in an abnormally large change in heart rate. This large and sudden change in heart rate results in light-headedness, blurry vision, or simply feeling weak. Other commonly associated conditions include irritable bowel disease, insomnia, and headaches. The average age of onset is twenty years old and it occurs more often in females.

'I had the kind of classic issue of POTS, which is you can't control your heart rate properly . . . and then your blood pressure drops . . . my digestive system wasn't working and then I had problems with my immune system and infections and then chronic fatigue . . . so I spent about six months or so in bed, just taking all these drugs and they just didn't have enough effect.'

As the medical options ran out, Ella did what many of us would do today; she asked the all-knowing Doctor Google.

'I started researching, like kinds of alternative things I could look at, and I came across lots of stories of people who'd used a change in diet and lifestyle to help manage all kinds of conditions, which I was – to be honest – incredibly sceptical of. It seemed quite bizarre to me that that could be an effective thing . . . but at this point . . . anything's worth a try, really.'

Many of these stories referenced a book called *The China Study*, which was billed as 'the most comprehensive study of nutrition ever conducted'. Crucially, it advocated a 'plant-based' diet for curing all manner of diseases. Ella, tired of being unwell, was readily convinced, and overnight she gave up meat, dairy, refined sugar, gluten and processed food. In the process of this drastic change in her diet, Ella ended up getting better. Ella started a food blog in 2012, to chart how she changed her diet to change her health, how she began to eat 'clean'; and thus Deliciously Ella was born. Ella had been dubbed in the media, much to her later annoyance, as 'The Queen of Clean'. It is true that Ella did not coin the term 'clean' for food. The writer Bee Wilson traces its first use in reference to a diet to Tosca Reno, a Canadian fitness model who published a book called *The Eat-Clean Diet*.[1] In it, Tosca describes her journey of how she lost 34kg (75lb). Thus in its first incarnation, 'clean' was really more of a weight-loss plan. Ella, however, already svelte, clearly did not have a weight problem; she was a model after all. Rather, Ella's story was one of changing her diet to cure herself, while eschewing conventional pharmaceutical solutions, and it has proven hugely influential. In her first eponymous book, *Deliciously Ella*, which was published in 2015, Ella opened with her own story of healing, thus powerfully framing everything that followed through its prism. As a result, what emerges is more than a book of vegan recipes, but a lifestyle; an instruction manual to eat 'clean' and be healthy like Ella; to eat like Ella and, dare I say, to look like Ella. None of this was explicitly stated of course; that would have been vulgar, and Ella was anything but. The implicit message, however, was at the forefront of her brand; it was very attractive and clearly in demand. *Deliciously Ella* sold 32,000 copies in its first week of release alone.

Prof T. Colin Campbell published *The China Study* in 2005 and in it he argued that the only truly safe way to eat was to follow a plant-based diet; he believed that there was no safe dose of animal-based protein. This message was eagerly devoured by certain sectors of society, including some very influential people. One such person was Bill Clinton, who in an effort to combat his heart disease, changed his diet after reading *The China Study*, as well as *Prevent and Reverse Heart Disease* by Caldwell Esselstyn. Caldwell Esselstyn and Colin Campbell became close friends, brought together by a common philosophy, and both of their books have become the foundational texts for the plant-based movement.

WHY PLANT-BASED AND NOT VEGAN?

I must admit that before I started researching for the documentary and for this book, I had not realised that there was a difference between being plant-based and vegan. When I made the mistake of using the term vegan while speaking to a group of people living a plant-based lifestyle, I got responses ranging from mild annoyance to outright aggression. People choose to be vegans for ethical reasons or environmental reasons or both. While I myself am not vegan, I can understand these reasons. Generally speaking, most plant-based dieters do not identify as vegans because of this (to quote one of the plant-based practitioners) 'baggage'. Folks who practise plant-based living, almost all of whom have been inspired by Campbell and Esselstyn, do so because they believe that animal-based protein will kill them. The motivation is therefore very different.

A plant-based diet is also more strict than a vegan diet. Food is considered vegan so long as it does not contain animal parts or derivatives. So a plant-based meal is in effect 'food from plants', and would clearly be suitable for vegans. However, while all plant-based food is vegan, the reverse is not true. There are all manner of processed foods that are free of animal products, but are not suitable for people sticking to a whole foods, plant-based diet. Examples include liquid calories such as soda, energy drinks and other sweetened beverages; refined foods such as those made with bleached flour and refined sugars; and foods containing chemical additives such as artificial colourings, flavourings and preservatives, including dairy-free pastries and low-calorie soda. This would mean that '*faux*-meat' products, such as those produced by Quorn or Linda McCartney, do not meet these criteria. There is a more extreme strain of 'plant-based' that I detail below, but broadly, to qualify as plant-based, the food has to, ostensibly, resemble the plant from which it came. I did look up to see if tofu was allowed, seeing that it is processed and does not resemble in anyway the source soybean. I was surprised (although I probably shouldn't have been) about the amount of discussion on this one point; but the consensus appears to be that while tofu is indeed processed, it is not 'too' processed, and is therefore acceptably plant-based. The other thing I looked up was whether or not mushrooms are plant-based. Mushrooms, you see, are in the kingdom 'Fungi' and are not members of either the Animalia or Plantae kingdom; so they are not actually plants at all. In lieu of an answer, I'll instead quote a user from a Reddit Plant-Based Diet forum, 'I wouldn't avoid them because of semantics. Mushrooms are awesome.' That was an awesome response, to which I have nothing more to add! But yes, mushrooms are 'plant-based', in spite of the semantics.

ALL THE T (COLIN CAMPBELL) IN CHINA

Colin Campbell's '*The China Study*' took its name from 'The China–Cornell–Oxford Project', a large observational population-based study looking at the incidence of disease in 1980s rural China. The lead researchers were Chen Junshi, of the Chinese

Academy of Preventive Medicine in Beijing, Li Junyao of the China Cancer Institute, Richard Peto of the University of Oxford, and T. Colin Campbell himself, who was from Cornell University in Ithaca, New York State. Colin and his colleagues gathered data from 6,500 people living in 65 different counties to try and understand the relationship between diet and health. This resulted in an 894-page tome, published in 1990, entitled *Diet, Life-Style, and Mortality in China: A Study of the Characteristics of 65 Chinese Counties*. I don't think I'm going out on a limb here by saying that while it was of interest to the epidemiological community, this book was not a page-turner that ended up on the *New York Times* bestseller list. But then again, as it was written as an academic text, it was not meant to. Then, in early 2005, Colin, together with his youngest son Thomas Campbell, introduced *The China Study* to the world. It was a publishing sensation that did capture the public imagination. However, in spite of taking its name from the China–Cornell–Oxford Project, a brief and select summary of the results only occupied one of the eighteen chapters in the book. Instead, Colin used it as the key piece of evidence to argue the benefits of a plant-based diet.

Whilst in the US for the *Clean Eating* documentary, I managed to interview Colin Campbell and Cladwell Esselstyn in Cleveland. Although Colin Campbell lived in upstate New York, he travelled often to visit Caldwell Esselstyn, who was based in Cleveland. Timing, as they say, is everything, and there emerged an unusual and valuable opportunity, to interview two of the most influential figures in the plant-based movement, on the same day.

I met with Colin at a fruit farm in Chesterland, a suburb of Cleveland. He was a spritely, silver-haired eighty-two-year-old (in 2016), slightly shorter than me and in fabulous shape. It was a sunny day in early autumn, the leaves were beginning to take on an amber hue, the pumpkins were just large enough for the Halloween harvest and the apples in the orchard were blushing red, begging to be picked. Speaking to Colin amongst the rows of apple trees laden with fruit was visually very striking; but clearly not striking enough for the producers, who thought it would add dynamism to the scene for me to conduct the interview whilst chauffeuring the professor around on a golf buggy. I'd just like to point out that driving around an apple orchard in an unfamiliar vehicle, whilst following another buggy carrying the film crew, and at the same time trying to interview Colin without the benefit of notes, required a significant proportion of my neurons to be firing effectively. Thank the good lord for coffee, I say; but I digress.

Colin's parents were dairy farmers, and *The China Study* opens in 1946 on the Campbell dairy farm, where a twelve-year-old Colin had just finished a breakfast of eggs, sausage and bacon washed down with whole milk, having been up since 4.30 a.m. helping his dad milk the cattle. Very quickly, we learnt that Colin's dad had his first heart attack at sixty-one, with a second, more serious, coronary event eventually killing him at the age of seventy.

'Now, after decades of doing experimental research on diet and health, I know that the very disease that killed my father, heart disease, can be prevented, even reversed . . . without life-threatening surgery and without potentially lethal drugs. I have learned that it can be achieved simply by eating the right food.'[2]

Then, in the very next section, Colin rapidly pivoted towards cancer. He provided some scary statistics from the American Cancer Society, that 47 per cent of American males and 38 per cent of American females would be diagnosed with some form of cancer during their lifetime. The numbers from Cancer Research UK were equally sobering, with 50 per cent of people in the UK born after 1960 likely to be diagnosed with cancer at some point. Then Colin said:

'Contrary to what many believe, cancer is not a natural event. Adopting a healthy diet and lifestyle can prevent the majority of cancers in the United States. Old age can and should be graceful and peaceful.'[3]

In a span of four paragraphs in Chapter 1, he clearly and succinctly set the foundation for everything that followed. First, Colin didn't believe in 'life-threatening' surgery and 'potentially lethal' drugs; which was of note, given that most of the tools available in conventional modern medicine were either pharmaceutical or surgical. Second, Colin believed that a healthy diet and lifestyle could prevent cancer and heart disease; in fact, as you read through the rest of the book, he believed that most, if not all diseases could be cured by diet and lifestyle. These were big and very attractive statements; you could see how someone like Ella was hooked. I mean, what sane person would want to age UNgracefully and UNpeacefully?

THE FUNGUS IN PEANUT BUTTER

Colin's journey from a young nutritional biochemist to *The China Study* began in the mid-1960s, when he joined a project in the Philippines called 'Mothercraft'. It was set up to educate the mothers of malnourished Filipino children about growing the right types of food, with the focus on increasing the amount of protein the children were eating. The strategy was to develop local crops of peanuts, which, like the soybean, was a nitrogen-fixing legume that was rich in protein. The problem at the time with peanuts was that they were often contaminated with a fungus that produced a toxin called aflatoxin, which at high doses had been shown to cause liver cancer in rats. As it turned out, in the Philippines, it wasn't the whole peanuts that had high levels of aflatoxin, rather it was peanut butter. This was because the best peanuts were hand selected off the production line to be sold as whole nuts, while the most mouldy and hence unattractive nuts were made into peanut butter. The two largest cities in the country, Manila and Cebu, had the highest rate of liver cancer, and Manila in particular consumed the most peanut butter and hence aflatoxin. And because children were the major consumers of peanut butter, they were the ones most susceptible to aflatoxin and its carcinogenic effects. Rates of childhood liver cancer in the Philippines were tragically high. Why is any of this relevant? Well, Colin was acquainted with a prominent Filipino doctor, Jose Caedo, who was an advisor to the then President Marcos. Dr Caedo, had observed (anecdotally I assume, because no numbers were provided) that the children getting the cancer appeared to be from the most well-off families, who were fed well and presumably had ready access to meat. Colin's conclusion from this observation was that the children getting the most protein had the highest rates of liver cancer. This was the first piece of the jigsaw.

'TURNING ON' CANCER

Back in the United States, Colin began some experiments on rats in order to see if he could model the Filipino liver-cancer observation. What he did was to treat rats with aflatoxin, which made them susceptible to getting cancer. He then wanted to see what would happen if he fed the rats different amounts of protein. He chose to use the milk protein casein. It was plentiful and I suppose cheaper than trying to feed chunks of beef to the rats (probably less smelly too). He gave one group of the aflatoxin-treated rats food containing 5 per cent casein, and another group food containing 20 per cent casein. Astonishingly, he found that all of the aflatoxin treated rats that were fed the 20 per cent casein ended up with liver cancer, whereas none of the rats on the 5 per cent casein diet got cancer. Was this true for other types of protein as well? How about plant-based protein? Colin tried the same experiment again, but this time with the wheat protein gluten and also soy protein; 20 per cent of either gluten or soy protein did not trigger liver cancer in aflatoxin-treated rats. Colin's conclusion from these set of experiments: animal-based protein (casein) could 'turn on' cancer, whereas plant-based protein (gluten and soy) did not.[4] This was the second piece of the jigsaw.

SIXTY-FIVE COUNTIES IN RURAL CHINA

In the early 1980s, Dr Chen Junshi, of the Chinese Academy of Preventive Medicine in Beijing, visited Colin's lab in Cornell University. It had been known since the late 1970s that in China cancer was geographically localised, with prevalence of certain cancers far higher in some places than others. Some of the differences were stark, with parts of the country having cancer rates 100 times higher than others. This was particularly striking because it occurred in a country where 87 per cent of the population were Han Chinese (as am I), so of the same ethnicity, and therefore relatively genetically homogeneous. Colin posed the question:

'Might it be possible that cancer is largely due to environmental/ lifestyle factors, and not genetics?'[5]

I feel that I have to interject with one of my 'genetics primers' here, to provide some perspective on this question. Cancer genetics is hideously complex. Inherited genetic mutations play a major role in about 5 to 10 per cent of all cancers, but these mutations are not 100 per cent 'penetrant'; meaning just because you carry the mutation doesn't mean you will get the disease. So, for example, if a woman carries a mutation in either the *BRCA1* or *BRCA2* genes, they will have a 40–85 per cent lifetime risk of getting breast cancer, versus a background risk of 12 per cent if they don't carry a mutation. Why is there a range and why is it not 100 per cent?

BRCA1 and *BRCA2* are both 'tumour suppressors', playing a role in repairing damaged DNA. Having a mutation in either of these genes is, in and of itself, not sufficient to result in cancer. What you need is a so-called 'second hit', another DNA-damaging mutation somewhere else, caused by an environmental insult. This can be radiation, or pollution, or smoking, or diet amongst many other things. DNA damage is happening all the time in all of us but (panic not) most of us have DNA repair enzymes, like the *BRCA* genes, to fix these problems as they happen. Carrying a mutation in one of the *BRCA* genes, or a few other tumour suppressor genes, makes you susceptible to cancer, because that DNA damage is not fixed. Sometimes (but not always) unrepaired DNA damage can turn a cell cancerous, meaning it begins to replicate uncontrollably. What about the other 90–95 per cent of cancers where genetic mutations don't play a major role? Does that mean that genes have no role to play in these cancers? Absolutely not! Everything about us has a genetic and an environmental component, and that includes our susceptibility to getting cancer. Many people, including even some of those who smoke, will never get cancer, because they are simply not genetically susceptible. For those who are susceptible, then your environment, whether or not you smoke, or how healthy or unhealthy your diet is, are all important influences on whether you end up getting cancer.

It was this question of trying to identify the environmental factors influencing cancer rates in China that motivated Colin and Dr Chen to set up the China–Cornell–Oxford Project, together with Li Junyao from the China Cancer Institute and Richard Peto of the University of Oxford. A total of 6,500 people living in 65 different rural counties in China were measured for 367 different variables, including anthropomorphic measures (height, weight etc.), blood lipid and cholesterol levels, prevalence of disease and diet. Given the geographic spread of the various counties it was, by any measure, a heroic effort. The team identified 'more than

8,000 statistically significant associations between lifestyle, diet and disease variables.'[6]

The headline association, the one Colin focussed relentlessly on, was that '... people who ate the most animal-based foods got the most chronic disease. Even relatively small intakes of animal-based food were associated with adverse effects.'[7] Thus, Colin concluded that 'whole plant-based foods were beneficial, and animal-based foods were not.'[8] This was the third and final piece of the jigsaw.

THE ONE DIET TO CURE ALL DISEASE . . .

With his Filipino experience, his rat casein experiments and then the China project, Colin had, in his mind, the complete picture, and took one final, very large, step. In the beginning of Part II of *The China Study*, he wrote:

'... the same diet that is good for the prevention of cancer is also good for the prevention of heart disease, as well as obesity, diabetes, cataracts, macular degeneration, Alzheimer's, cognitive dysfunction, multiple sclerosis, osteoporosis and other diseases. Furthermore, this diet can benefit everyone, regardless of his or her genes or personal dispositions ... there is only one diet to counteract all of these diseases: a whole food, plant-based diet.'[9]

The one diet to cure all disease, in everyone, regardless of their genetic background. From this one statement has emerged the whole plant-based movement.

. . . OR IS IT?

However, the scientific foundations upon which *The China Study* is built were not as stable as they seemed. Over the past decade, there have been some forensically detailed (I am not exaggerating) critiques of Colin Campbell's opus,[10] for those who enjoy their prose sprinkled with a healthy dose of tables, graphs and statistics. Fear not, that is not my intention here. I just want to raise some of the major concerns about Colin's interpretation of the data, and how he uses it to argue that there is no safe dose of animal protein.

THE LEAST LIKELY EXPLANATION

Let's begin with the observation from the Philippines that it was the most well-off children that were having the highest rates of cancer. Colin formed the conclusion that this was the case because they were likely to have been fed more meat than poorer children. Colin was probably correct that children from richer families ate more meat. However, he completely ignored all of the other possible factors that were associated with being more well off. For example, the better-off children could have been living in the larger cities and therefore been subject to more pollution; perhaps they were being driven around more, and therefore had less exercise; or being more well-off could have also meant greater access to refined carbohydrates or high sugar or higher-fat food. Any combination of these factors could have explained the higher rates of cancer. In fact, there was no reason to believe that eating more meat was the most likely explanation.

PROTEIN IS PROTEIN

How convincing were the experiments showing that casein 'turned on' cancer in rats? I don't doubt Colin's results as he presented them. I just question the logic of jumping from powdered casein and equating it to all animal protein. In fact Colin himself, together with a graduate student, Tom O'Connor, published a paper showing that fish protein mixed with fish oil (one might accept this to be a facsimile of 'fish'), as compared to fish protein mixed with corn oil (this would not be 'fish'), had the potential to act as inhibitory agents in cancer development.[11] This completely contradicted his own argument that ALL animal-based protein could 'turn on' cancer. What of the fact that the plant-based proteins gluten and soy tested by Colin did not induce cancer? All proteins are made up of a mix of twenty different building blocks called 'amino acids'. Gluten, as it turns out, is deficient in one particular amino acid called lysine. In yet another paper published by Colin, which wasn't included in *The China Study*, he showed that when you used gluten supplemented with lysine, it behaved exactly like casein to induce cancer in rats.[12] In other words, there was nothing special about casein because it came out of a cow that made it able to 'turn on' cancer in the very restrictive conditions tested by Colin. Plant-based gluten did the very same thing, as long as a little bit of lysine was sprinkled in to make it a 'complete' protein.

POWER AND PROXY

And finally, how about the third of Colin's three pillars, the China project? First, in terms of the number of measurements taken, the project was not actually as well 'powered' as it initially seemed. With 6,500 people from 65 different counties, on average, 100 people were studied per county; surely that sounds like a lot? Well yes, except that the measurements from each county, in particular those from blood, were aggregated; meaning that the 100 blood samples from each county were pooled into a large volume before being analysed. If we take the measurement of blood cholesterol levels as an example, this pooling resulted in only 65 different cholesterol levels (one from each county), as opposed to 6,500 different cholesterol levels (100 from each county).

If you had 100 different cholesterol levels from each county, you could have examined the spread of the data, and seen if everyone from each county had roughly the same measurements, or were there a few unusual individuals with very high or very low levels skewing the data? In essence, the aggregation of samples resulted in a huge loss of statistical 'power', which in turn reduced the confidence of whether a particular level of cholesterol was truly representative for that county; whether cholesterol levels were actually different between counties; or whether cholesterol levels were associated with any of the other 366 measurements that were taken.

Which takes us nicely to the second point. Of the 'more than 8,000 statistically significant associations between lifestyle, diet and disease variables', Colin, like a laser beam, focussed on meat intake in each county, and its association with disease. Except that, instead of using the actual amount of meat eaten (averaged for each county) in his association studies, he used cholesterol levels as a proxy instead. What does this mean exactly? Well, the China project data did show that higher cholesterol levels are positively associated with various cancers. It also showed that higher cholesterol levels are associated with increased intake of meat. Colin thus made the conclusion, via an indirect connection, using cholesterol as a proxy, that higher intake of meat was linked to cancer. But, and it was a very big but, if you compare meat intake directly with different cancers, there are as many negative correlations as there are positive ones, with none of them reaching statistical significance. Why? Because cholesterol levels are affected by all kinds of factors, not just meat intake. In particular, genetics play a big role in influencing cholesterol levels, independent of how much meat or fat or even plants you might consume.

There are many other criticisms that have been levelled at *The China Study*. But the fact of the matter was while higher cholesterol levels (with all the caveats that come with the aggregation of data) were associated with increased incidence of cancers, the data in the China project did not actually show any significant associations between meat intake and disease.

NOTHING WITH A MOTHER OR A FACE

My conversation with Colin in the orchard had gone on for a lot longer than expected, and as a consequence we were now late for our visit with Caldwell Esselstyn. Colin kindly agreed to ride along with me, this time in a rented black Ford Mustang convertible (I was really getting into driving those Mustangs!), so he could direct me the 10 miles or so to Esselstyn's home.

Caldwell B. Esselstyn Jr. (everyone simply calls him Ess) is a former surgeon at the Cleveland Clinic. He is also, impressively, an Olympic gold medallist in rowing from the 1956 Melbourne games, and was awarded the Bronze Star as an army surgeon in Vietnam. As Colin and I got out of the car, we were greeted by Ess's wife Ann. Ann was a larger-than-life character, a delightful force of nature. At that very moment, however, she was none too pleased with us; we were nearly two hours late after all, so it was entirely understandable and I was very apologetic. As we walked into the house, we were greeted by a cacophony of noise. Ann and Ess had invited their family along with three of Ess's patients to meet me and the crew; it was a veritable party! Ess was essentially the same age as Colin, eighty-three years old when I met him that day in 2016. He was very tall, and although lanky now, I could see that he would have been quite the physical specimen during his rowing years.

In 2007, Ess wrote *Prevent and Reverse Heart Disease*, which claimed, emblazoned on the front cover, to provide a 'revolutionary, scientifically proven, nutrition-based cure' to heart disease [13]

His programme was simple, austere and, by any measure, very extreme:

- You may not eat anything with a mother or a face (no meat, poultry or fish)
- You cannot eat dairy products
- You must not consume oil of any kind – not a drop (not even olive oil)
- Generally you cannot eat nuts or avocados.

Wow. This is really taking plant-based to a whole other level; it is the only diet I know of that prohibits olive oil, nuts and avocados! Of note, Ess only removed (non-fat) dairy products from the list of allowable foods after reading *The China Study*, and Campbell only removed oil from his diet after meeting Ess. Both Colin and Ess appeared together in an independently produced documentary, *Forks over Knives*, which was released in 2011, in which both the China Project and Ess's work, as well as the benefits of this diet, featured prominently. Hence, many have taken to calling this extreme plant-based diet the *Forks over Knives* diet, in contrast to a more conventional (a loosely used term here) plant-based diet.

Ess's claim that this extreme diet was 'scientifically proven' came from his own publication in 1995, where he concluded:

'A physician can influence patients in the decision to adopt a very low-fat diet that, combined with lipid-lowering drugs, can reduce cholesterol levels . . . and uniformly result in the arrest or reversal of coronary artery (heart) disease.'[14]

If you read the paper, however, two major problems emerge. First, the study was not controlled. Ess's original intent was to have one group of patients on the diet and another receiving standard cardiac care and then compare how the two groups had fared after three years. This is known as a randomised controlled trial, and is the 'gold standard' for testing the effectiveness of an intervention.

Unfortunately this approach, due to a 'lack of funding, was not practical'.[14] Instead, 24 patients, all suffering from heart disease, began the study, and all were placed on the extreme plant-based diet. Six patients ended up dropping out because they could not tolerate the diet (you could imagine how much fun it would have been), leaving 18 highly motivated people in the study. Second, there were two major confounding factors. All patients were on cholesterol-lowering medications and half of the remaining patients had already undergone surgery for their heart condition. So while the group of 18 did tremendously well in the study, because of the lack of a control group and all of the confounding factors, it was impossible to know if the diet had anything to with their outcome.

While at Ess's house, I took the opportunity to interview three of his patients whom he had successfully treated. They were two men and a woman, all in their forties or fifties, looking happy and well, and very eager to share their stories. All had undoubtedly received a new lease of life under Ess's care, so I was keen to speak to them. What became abundantly clear just a few minutes into our conversation, was that all three had lost a tremendous amount of weight, ranging from 15–21 kilograms (33–46 pounds). One of the men told me, 'I have lost so much weight, that I can now exercise again! I can walk the dog, garden, even go for a jog!'

There was, it turned out, a third major confounding factor. Because of the very restrictive diet, certainly the most extreme examined in this book, most people who stuck to it ended up losing a huge amount of weight. Vegetables, fruits, legumes and whole grains, which are pretty much all you can eat on this diet, all have very low caloric availability, and there is only so much time in the day you can spend eating and therefore only so many calories you can absorb. As I discussed in Chapter 5, many diseases including type 2 diabetes, heart disease and certain cancers, are linked to obesity. As a result, losing a large amount of weight reverses type 2 diabetes in most (but not all) people and tremendously reduces the risk for heart disease and some cancers.

Thus, the most likely explanation for the miraculous health improvements that Ess saw in his patients after they went on an extreme plant-based diet was because they lost large amounts of weight, rather than because of the removal of animal protein and fat *per se*. On top of that, as a result of the weight loss, they became more mobile and active, which independent of weight loss would have provided metabolic and cardiovascular benefits.

AS IF I HAD ALL THE EVIDENCE

Towards the end of my interview with Colin, I asked him:

'... I guess my question is, when you give nutritional advice, which is quite extreme, by asking to remove an entire food group...'

Colin quickly interrupted me with his reply:

'... I never. What I say, this is the goal. And the reason I say it's the goal, is not because we have all the science in ... I just simply say, this is the goal, because as we proceed in that direction, I don't see any harm occurring. So I'm not making more arguments that, you know, as if I had all the evidence, all the empirical evidence, to say this is true for everyone, I'm not saying that. I'm simply saying that ... this idea here ... is far greater in terms of the contribution to human health, than any other idea I know.'

In other words, Colin himself admitted that he didn't have the evidence that being plant-based was the *only* safe way to eat.

ASSOCIATION VS CAUSATION

What about Ella, though? Why did her POTS go away after she shifted to a plant-based diet? Ella was always lean, so it couldn't have been down to weight loss. While the causes of POTS are poorly understood, more than 50 per cent of people whose condition was triggered by a viral infection get better within five years. Additionally 90 per cent of POTS sufferers improve with treatment. In all likelihood, Ella would have got better anyway, whether or not she embraced a plant-based diet. But embrace it she did, and Ella has, quite understandably, associated her improvement in health with her change in diet. The question is, did her shift in diet *cause* her health to improve? It may or may not have helped; we will never know, because a proper study was not conducted. But I do believe that if changing her diet made her feel better, then it was the right thing for her to do. It doesn't, however, mean that it is the right thing for everyone to do.

POST-TRUTH & PHARMA GILES

Colin Campbell and Caldwell Esselstyn both began their careers as men of science; Colin a professor in Biochemistry and Ess a surgeon. Yet at some point, they moved away from their scientific roots and entered, embraced even, the world of evangelism. Their followers at the more extreme end of the plant-based movement take on 'non-believers' with evangelical zeal. No, I do not believe that I am engaging in hyperbole. The rules, after all, must be followed. This explains their annoyance with vegans, because they are not doing it in the 'right' way or for the 'right' reasons.

After the *Clean Eating* documentary aired in the UK on the

19th January 2016, I was attacked vociferously, online, by plant-based zealots for my evidence-based views. This was driven in large part by Colin Campbell, who accused me of being funded by 'big pharma' and therefore having a vested interest in advocating that a dietary approach does not work, so that I can sell pills. For the record, I am an employee of the University of Cambridge, and the vast majority of my research is funded by the UK Medical Research Council, which is a government funding body. My research interest is in trying to understand the genetics and mechanisms underlying obesity, so that we can effectively tackle the obesity problem. I'm not in the business of selling pills. So this accusation was demonstrably untrue.

In this 'post-truth' world, none of the plant-based zealots would be swayed. To them, I remained a carnivorous drug-company shill. I heard about it for weeks and weeks after, with incessant trolling coming through on Facebook, Instagram and, in particular, Twitter. Someone dug out my CV from somewhere and compared it to Colin's. Another even made a 15-minute video attacking me that was viewed tens of thousands of times, until it was pulled down for using copyrighted material. Because it was my first time experiencing the full wrath of trolls, it was all just a little bit shocking. However, I now understood this was what I should expect when sticking my head above the parapet. Another presenter at the BBC told me 'if you're not being trolled, then you aren't doing it right'.

BACK TO THE AMBUSH

The advice that I was given by the BBC was not to engage. Let them shout, let them seethe and let them rage, but do not engage, and they would eventually tire. The BBC were right. About a month after it all began, it gradually quietened down, and my Twitter account became mine again.

Until nine months later at 'Food Matters Live', when I found myself ambushed by that plant-based zealot.

If you had access to the footage, I reckon you could tell from my eyes when I realised I'd been had. In my head, I was running through my options. I could have stood up and walked away . . . but seeing as there was a camera on me, they would have used the clip of me refusing to participate in a debate. All right then, if this was an ambush, then so be it; I didn't have any other choice but to lock horns and engage. It clearly wasn't a debate, though, because he regurgitated questions that came from Colin's letter of complaint; so it was nothing I hadn't heard before, and I simply responded to all of the questions. When he realised he wasn't going to get anything new out of me, he kept asking me variations of the same question over and over again.

'Are you not an unchangeable carnivore with an anti-plant-based agenda?'

At this point, I felt the interview was over. I stood up, thanked the interviewer, and walked away.

IS MEAT BAD FOR YOU?

So, is meat bad for you? Well, here is where the rubber hits the road. It all depends on what type of meat we are talking about and how it is prepared. In a paper published in *Lancet Oncology*,[15] the International Agency for Research on Cancer (IARC) reviewed over 800 different published epidemiological studies looking at the links between red and processed meat and cancer. The evidence for processed meat, which included bacon (nooooo!), sausages and ham, increasing your risk of cancer was pretty powerful. While the exact reasons for this have yet to be nailed down, the nitrite preservatives are very likely to play a significant role. IARC found an 18 per cent (!) increase in risk of colorectal cancer if you ate

50 grams of processed meat every day. That is about three rashers of bacon or one sausage per day. That does sound scary, but the 18 per cent does not refer to absolute risk, rather to relative risk. The life-time 'absolute' risk of colorectal cancer is 5 per cent. An 18 per cent increase in relative risk means your lifetime 'absolute' risk goes up to 5.9 per cent. Look, I'm not saying that this is great news, but it is important to understand the actual numbers. Let's compare this with smoking. According to Cancer Research UK, smoking three cigarettes a day increases your risk of lung cancer by six times . . . which is a 600 per cent increase. Smoking 20 cigarettes a day increases your likelihood of getting cancer by 2,600 per cent (not a typo)![16] With these numbers, it doesn't matter what your absolute risk is! So processed meat increases risk of cancer, but one has to keep things in perspective. This is currently the most powerful evidence linking an animal-based protein to cancer.

Red meat is next on the list, but to quote the *Lancet Oncology* paper:

'Chance, bias, and confounding could not be ruled out with the same degree of confidence for the data on red meat consumption, since no clear association was seen in several of the high-quality studies and residual confounding from other diet and lifestyle risk is difficult to exclude. The Working Group concluded that there is limited evidence in human beings for the carcinogenicity of the consumption of red meat.'

Translating that into English, what IARC are trying to say is that some studies show a risk, while others don't.

The consensus from the literature indicates that a moderate intake (200g/day) of white meat, such as chicken and turkey, shows no increased risk, whereas there appears to be a beneficial effect of fish (I will discuss this in Chapter 11). The American Cancer Society (ACS), Cancer Research UK, the British Heart Foundation and the UK NHS advice regarding meat is to *'Minimise your intake of processed meats such as bacon, sausage, lunch meats, and hot dogs. Choose fish, poultry, or beans instead of red meat (beef, pork, and lamb). If you eat red meat, choose lean cuts and eat smaller portions.*[17]

A FIRST WORLD PROBLEM

It should be no surprise that *The China Study* and *Prevent and Reverse Heart Disease* have been so widely embraced within the plant-based community. After all, it provides a 'scientific' rationale for avoiding all animal foods. It is a validation of their lifestyle; it is a confirmation of their bias.

In reality, one has to be in a privileged position in order to follow such a restrictive diet. To worry about eating avocados, olive oil, nuts, fish, chicken, milk and eggs. Really? It is a first-world problem. If you and your family were malnourished, your first priority would be to get food, any food. Milk and eggs are cheap and very nutrient dense, and clearly the availability of any meat at all would be welcome. And what is anyone supposed to do about finding a replacement for avocados? How are you supposed to make guacamole without avocados? What is life without guacamole after all?

I have absolutely nothing against people choosing to eat in a plant-based or vegan fashion. There are well catalogued issues with micronutrient deficiencies, in particular vitamin B12, which is found largely in animal-based products, and iodine.[18] One also has to be careful getting enough protein that covers the full spectrum of amino acids. But as long as it is done properly and these deficiencies are met, then it is a healthy way to live. It is a choice. It is a choice that we are privileged enough to have the opportunity to make. Do we, the privileged, eat too much meat? Undoubtedly so. It is a problem and it is something we will have to address. That does not mean that a modest amount of animal-based protein is bad for you; in fact most evidence indicates it is likely to be beneficial. I have already mentioned that in 2014, there were an estimated 8.4 million people in the UK, the world's 6th largest economy, living in households reporting having insufficient food, the equivalent of the entire population of London or New York. They don't have the luxury to try and find plant-based options when animal-based protein, in moderation, does no harm; when olive oil and nuts do absolutely no harm. Suggesting that any and all animal-based protein is harmful, while many people in the world are not getting enough nutritious food is not based on any reliable scientific evidence; it is pseudoscience.

CHAPTER 8

Cleanse and detox

The Shoreditch Grind is a cylindrical charcoal-coloured brick building, with a recording studio on the second floor and a trendy café/restaurant/cocktail bar below. It sits on the Old Street round-about in central London, right next to the Underground station. It was early spring, near the end of March in 2016. The traffic on the roundabout was just beginning to build towards rush hour, but was not yet heavy enough to be unpleasant, and the late-afternoon sun made it just warm enough to contemplate sitting outside. I ordered myself a beer, an American style IPA, and sat down. I had just taken my first glug from the bottle, when the person I was waiting for walked up to the table.

'Giles? Hi, I'm Sarah!'

Sarah Jordan was Canadian (what's not to love about a country with a maple leaf on their flag?), tall and almost lanky (she used to be a high jumper), strikingly good-looking (she used to be a model), was fluent in both English and French (*enchantée*) and a biochemistry undergraduate at King's College in London on her way to a first-class degree. If the universe was in anyway fair, she should have been exceedingly annoying, but she wasn't. We had not met in person before, but I guess chrome-dome Chinese guys hanging out and trying to fit in at the Shoreditch Grind were few and far between.

Sarah had contacted me by email a few weeks before, looking for a summer placement in my lab. Unfortunately, the inn was full, and there was no way I could accommodate her. I was going to turn her down outright, but something made me tell her about my book project, which I was researching at the time, and I ended up asking Sarah if she would like to help me with research for the book. Much to my surprise, she said yes almost immediately. Sarah told me that she had tried more diets, 'detox' and 'cleanse' programmes than she would like to admit. She had tried fasting around the full moon, eating bentonite clay and 'oil pulling' daily over the course of many months. She used to drink green juices and smoothies (sometimes multiple glasses or bottles a day), eat all kinds of plant-based 'super foods', so much so she was often mistaken for a vegan (she was not).

'I am also not an expert on nutrition, or bodily detoxification processes or a bona-fide scientist for that matter either. But having worked as a model, then a manager of a cold-pressed juice bar and now a student of biomedical sciences, I feel I have gained some insight into the health-food industry from pretty distinct vantage points.'

Oh wow. I had unknowingly found myself a juice bar-managing, smoothie-chugging, detox cleanse ex-model turned student of science. I had myself a bona-fide defector, an informant. I had my insider. We had to meet!

HELP SUSTAIN AN UNSUSTAINABLE STATE

I bought her a drink and we began to talk.

Sarah first came across cleansing and detox programmes where most other trends often start: the fashion industry. Working as a model in New York, juice cleanses and other fad diets were as pervasive as post-workout selfies and designer handbags or shoes or other illicit habits. Wherever you were in the city, rest assured there would nearly always be a cold-pressed juice bar within walking distance.

'I was never a fan of "the cleanse" *per se*, but because I was a little on the "curvy" side for a model, my diet was heavy on the liquids and vegetables, which were low in calories but still contained enough nutritional value for me to convince myself I wasn't depriving my body entirely.'

OMG, if Sarah was considered a little on the curvy side, I swear there was no hope for the rest of us.

'Having grown out of my prepubescent frame and constantly fighting my widened hips, I would incessantly research the benefits of various "super foods", looking for the magic ingredient that would help sustain an unsustainable state.'

Help sustain an unsustainable state . . . this was all great stuff. Note taking was not my forte, but I was scribbling furiously.

Cold-pressed green juices and smoothies were some of those magical products that promised to help maintain Sarah's figure, and thus her livelihood. They also conveniently fitted her criteria of being liquid and mostly plant-based. She was hardly unique in this and saw her peers go through extreme pre-Fashion Week preparation by undertaking various cleanses to 'lean out' already lean figures, under the pretence of losing weight 'the healthy way'. Sarah had obtained most of her information from various health-food blogs, the actual companies selling the stuff, or by word of mouth, typically from other equally ill-informed models, equally desperate to remain (ridiculously and unhealthily) thin and thus keep their jobs. In addition to fairly obsessive behaviour and mistrust in her body's ability to maintain itself, she developed some far-out ideas about how the body processed food and tried to abide by the many rules she had made up to ensure she kept her fragile systems in check. Sarah was lifting the lid and allowing me a first-hand peek into the industry, and she was not painting a pretty picture.

GET WITH THE CLEANSE PROGRAMME

While the first use of the term 'clean' in food can be traced to Tosca Reno (the Canadian fitness model who published the book *The Eat-Clean Diet*), its initial incarnation was really more of a weight-loss plan, as opposed to it cleaning or curing anything. Then along came the exotically named Alejandro Junger. A cardiologist by training, the Uruguayan-born, Los Angeles-based Junger introduced the concept of 'clean detox' to the world, revolutionising and colouring what both words mean to most of us today. He caught the eye of the actress Gwyneth Paltrow, who in 2008 praised Junger's approach on her newly launched lifestyle website GOOP. In 2009, Junger published *Clean: The Revolutionary Program to Restore the Body's Natural Ability to Heal Itself*, which became a bestseller. To this day, Junger continues to act as an advisor to Gwyneth Paltrow and GOOP.

The basic premise to 'cleanse and detox' is that throughout your life you build up toxins in your body, as a direct result of what you eat and drink, and how you live and breathe; toxins which you need to periodically purge from your body, to ensure and enable its healthy and correct functioning. It borrows heavily from the *faux*-Eastern philosophy of aligning one's body with one's spirit in order to attain inner peace and happiness, and in this instance, inner health.

If you peruse Junger's 'clean program' webpage (other detox programmes are available), you will see that the headline product is his 21-Day Cleanse Diet Program, designed by a medical doctor no less (Junger himself, I presume, although he is not so vulgar as to explicitly say so). He claims that typical benefits include 'improvements in skin, sleep, digestion, energy, healthy weight loss, and mental clarity with a reduction in bloating, constipation, headaches, and joint pain.'[1] His is a five-step process:

1) First you need to '*allow your body to heal itself*'; from all of the damage that has accumulated through living, I guess. He prescribes two liquid meals a day in the form of shakes (vanilla and chocolate to choose from), to 'streamline the digestive process' and 'reduce digestive load', so as to clean the slate to start afresh.

2) You have 'to *limit common allergy and inflammatory foods*'. Because, of course, there are many foods out there that 'can cause a build-up of mucus, fat, and inflammation in our bodies' (if there was a camera pointed to my face as I write this, you would see my deeply sceptical look on display . . . I have a terrible poker face). What are some of these awful foods? Well, they include caffeine and alcohol (OK, Dr Junger, you've lost me already), dairy and eggs, sugar, all vegetables in the *Solanaceae* or 'nightshade' family (potatoes, tomatoes, aubergines [eggplant], bell-peppers and chillies amongst many others) and red meat, which apparently causes a build-up of acids in the body (a big no-no; I tackle the myth of acidity and alkalinity in detail in Chapter 9), amongst other foods.

3) You have to try and '*get the most out of your food*'. We are of course surrounded by processed foods and quick options that aren't always the best for us. But, as I discuss in Chapter 4, what type of 'process' really does matter. Cooking is a process; fermentation is a process; curing is a process – the devil is in the detail. Junger says that his programme focusses on '*clean eating with a solid foundation of fruits, veggies, natural proteins, and healthy grains [which] unlocks our body's best state of being*.' Here is where the meatballs meet the sauce. What does Junger mean by 'clean eating'? In this context, he means that some foods, because of their very nature, will 'cleanse' you. By inference, this also means that other foods will 'dirty' you.

4) Junger talks about the importance of a '*12-Hour Window*'. He says that by leaving 12 hours between our last meal the day before and our breakfast, we are 'sending the signal to go into deep detox mode'; to let our body know that 'from 8 p.m. to 8 a.m., it's time to clean house'. I personally call this time 'sleep', but maybe that's just me.

5) Finally, all you have to do is to '*put it all together*', to 'create the perfect environment to start fresh'.

This 21-day programme is available to you at a snip, for USD$475! What a deal! Sadly, I don't think it currently ships outside the US.

But the 21 days are just a beginning of course. After the initial detoxification period, Junger then advises very cautiously reintroducing 'toxic triggers' such as wheat (the boogeyman) and dairy (the acidic boogeyman). This confused me slightly, because if they are so toxic, why reintroduce them at all? He also offers a maintenance kit of 'natural' powdered shakes and 'essential supplements'. I'm not sure how 'natural' powdered shakes and supplements in a pill really are, but there we go. He claims these will aid digestion, help maintain a healthy weight, promote hair growth (gosh, maybe I should look into these) and relieve skin conditions, as well as reduce anxiety, depression and mood swings. Rest assured, all of these products are, naturally, non-GMO, gluten-free, dairy-free, soy-free and nut-free. Wow, USD$138 buys you a lot . . . well, at the very least it will buy you about 30 days of maintenance, or around a month's-worth of keeping all of those toxins out. And before you ask, I did the maths for you; it means that maintaining your insides squeaky clean the Junger way will set you back USD$1,656 a year. Surely you are worth it?

A MODEL EXAMPLE

Sarah grew up on the Canadian prairies in a small city called Lloydminster, bordering the provinces of Alberta and Saskatchewan. To most people (well, to me anyway), Canada brings to mind the Rocky Mountains and evergreens, moose and grizzly bears, men wearing plaid shirts and funny hats while wielding axes and taking their aggression out on trees, and other such majestic, great-outdoorsy sights and sounds. Growing up on the prairies (did Sarah live in a little house? Did she call her dad 'Pa'?) offered a different topography, one that was bare and flat (it is said, in Saskatchewan, you can watch your dog run away for three days), and freezing most of the year. Despite the frigid temperatures and lack of much (any?) cultural activity, Sarah had a very busy youth dedicated mostly to dance and sport. She came from athletic stock and so athletic pursuits were a major focus in her family. Her sport of choice, in part because of her body geometry and in part because it didn't involve too much hand/eye coordination and because she was a little lazy and only had to run/jog/saunter nine paces, was the high jump. She was very good at getting her lanky frame over the bar and competed at a national and international level up until the age of seventeen, at which point she no longer enjoyed it and went into early athletic retirement.

Sarah then ended up in Montreal to attend university, where she began modelling part-time while she studied. Like many other young women of that age, this was when her body started to change. Her metabolism was no longer that of a fifteen-year old athlete, and she tried desperately to hold-off the 'freshman 15' (or the freshers' 14 here in the UK; in reference to the number of pounds an average first-year student in university gains after flying the nest) by adopting strange eating habits. Sarah had only just completed her first year when opportunities came a-knocking. She decided to put university on hold, and started modelling full time, while she had youth and body habitus on her side. Her 'mother agency' (that is, the primary agency that acts to manage a model's career and place them with agencies in other cities) was on board with her plan, but she was asked to 'get into shape' in order for it to fully work out. Sarah moved to New York, and her struggle to stay within the 'acceptable size range' for models began. She would cut out all bread and many grains, go on extreme diets before any work trip and work out incessantly. She modelled full time for around five years, before growing tired of the industry and quitting – having recognised her behaviour as being fairly obsessive and not sustainable.

WHAT IS A COLD-PRESSED JUICE CLEANSE?

At twenty-three years old, and now a steely-eyed veteran of the modelling industry, Sarah moved from New York to London. She wanted to return to university, this time to study science, but needed a job before her application was accepted and her course would begin. She started working for a shiny and new, super-clean, cold-pressed juice bar start-up that had recently opened its first location. She became the manager of the shop and would also speak at various workshops they hosted, promoting whatever they were selling. Being completely unqualified in every way to give dietary advice, Sarah had to navigate the many health concerns of her customers (which most people were surprisingly happy to divulge to their friendly cold-pressed juice sales-women). She would then 'prescribe' a juice that would relieve whatever was ailing them.

Each product normally came with some kind of health claim, depending on its ingredients. When customers asked about the benefits of each juice, Sarah would then rattle off a few buzz words to help them choose; she would, in essence, pitch each juice combo. Anything spicy, for instance, would increase metabolism, while anything green was detoxing, alkalising and good for weight loss. If a customer wanted something better for digestion, then ginger was the way to go; whereas if inflammation was a problem, then a dose of juiced pineapple would sort that out.

No one can argue that vegetable juice doesn't pack a lot of nutrients and isn't healthy for you. But does it balance the pH of the blood, clear up your skin and cure cancer?

'I can attest to the misinformation often spread for the sake of making a sale,' Sarah told me.

What exactly is cold-pressed juice? Well, instead of using a centrifugal juicer (the kind you would have in your own kitchen), which employs a blade that can heat up, cold pressing essentially squashes and squeezes the fruit and veg to remove their juices. The process is carried out in a giant fridge at 4°C which, so they say, ensures that the juice retains its highest possible nutritional density and 'enzymatic activity', while limiting oxidisation. It also allowed the juice to stay consumable for up to three days after pressing and so be bottled and sold in brightly coloured shops by tall, lanky women who used to model, and young men with six-pack abs. Some companies would then high-pressure-pasteurise the bottled juice which extended the shelf life to months. However, this process was frowned upon by the true raw-cold-pressed-green juice aficionados. Most juice companies are adamant about cold-pressing and tout it as being the optimal process for extracting juice (which has the added benefit of allowing them to charge £6 in the UK for the pleasure for a 500ml bottle – quite a lot of money).

The biggest and best sale for any juice company however, was the cleanse programme. The programme sold by Sarah, for example, cost around £40 a day for six juices and/or flavoured nut milks (dude, please), making the Junger programme look positively economical in comparison. For those of you not in the know (and I only know because Sarah told me), a 'juice cleanse' normally involves forgoing all solid foods, and instead ingesting around 3 litres of juice, containing 800–1,200 calories, a day, for a period ranging from one to seven days (or longer). The claim, made by the companies themselves, along with countless blogs, health gurus, celebrities and social-media stars, is that juice cleansing allows the liver, stomach and intestines to take a much-needed rest. The benefits of this are pretty much endless and include: improved digestion and metabolism, increased energy levels, weight loss, alkalisation of the blood, brightening of the skin, improved sleep and immune function, amplified detoxification processes, enhanced mental capacities, improved relationships, connecting deeper to your spiritual side and discovering the healthiest version of yourself. I mean, come on! Sign me up for the full seven-day programme!

Many people experience side-effects, including light-headedness, headaches, fatigue, cravings, pain and irritability. Contrary to any other time you are experiencing these symptoms, feeling awful is apparently supposed to be a good thing as it means that your body was super-toxic and is processing an increased load of those impurities. To quote directly from one company: 'A cold-pressed juice heals, nourishes and regenerates your whole body, helping to release toxins and rid the body of built-up waste.'[2] I for one experience the aforementioned feelings on a nearly daily basis, when I am late getting dinner into the oven by like five minutes after I cycle back from work and feel like I am starving to death. Little did I know that it was doing me good! And the bonus is that I get to feel like that without shelling out £40/day.

This marketing strategy is incredibly effective, with the juice cleansing business worth upwards of \$5 billion (£3.6 billion) per year. And of course it is! Who doesn't want the perfect skin, svelte body and seemingly glamourous life of those that undertake and endorse these programmes (the hiring of Sarah to manage the bar and sell the cleanses is a case in point)? In addition to celebrity and social-media 'influencer' testimonials, the companies further justify these huge claims by having 'reliable' doctors (I'm looking at you, Dr Junger) and other professionals backing them up.

YOUR LIVER IS WORTH IT

This seems to be an appropriate time to introduce one of the more underappreciated organs that keeps the body ticking. Our liver.

The liver plays a major role in carbohydrate, protein and lipid metabolism. For example, it converts glucose to glycogen when glucose levels are high, and converts glycogen back to glucose when glucose levels are low. It makes protein and it degrades protein. It is responsible for the synthesis of cholesterol, lipids and fatty acids. The liver also plays a key role in digestion through the production of bile, which is critical in the breakdown of fat, and in the storage of certain vitamins (A, D, B12 & K) and minerals (iron and copper). Crucially, and relevant to this chapter, our liver is responsible for the breakdown and excretion of many waste products. It is, in effect, a professional detox organ. The entire blood supply from our digestive tract and most other organs drains directly into the portal vein, which is piped straight into the liver. The liver then sorts through everything in the blood, storing or metabolising nutrients and working to eliminate toxins through a complex series of enzymatic processes. The first of these steps is to neutralise or alter the toxin. The next step is to take the altered toxin and alter it some more, often by adding another component to it such as a particular amino acid or sulphur. This renders the compound less harmful and often makes it water-soluble, thus it is able to be excreted from the system either in urine or bile. A healthy functioning liver does this all of the time, whether you're asleep or awake. It works harder after you've eaten, and after you've had a beer or a glass of wine. If you've had a few too many jars to drink, the blood then needs to pass through the liver a few times before the alcohol is metabolised, during which time you will feel its woozy effects. The liver is so effective in metabolising potential toxins that when drugs are being developed, the effective dose has to take into account the liver's 'drug-metabolism' rate.

The situation in which actual *bona-fide* 'detoxification' is needed is when someone is being treated for a dangerous level of a substance that is life-threatening. The term detox, for instance, is correctly used for the process of trying to remove drugs of abuse from your system; so going 'cold turkey'. But that is a process where you stop taking something, and then let your body, mostly your liver, clear out the drugs or chemicals that are in the system. Equally, many of you might have participated in 'dry January', where you try and give your liver 'a break' from all that festive champagne and port. Once again, this is a completely legitimate process, because you are giving up alcohol for a month. So exclusion is the way to do 'detox' because you are letting your liver get on with its professional role. There is no evidence that anything you eat can accelerate or enhance this process.

If something goes wrong with the liver, however (see below), thus hindering the physiological 'detoxing' that happens in the background all of the time, then things rapidly go south. The liver, together with your kidneys, intestines, lungs, lymphatic system and skin work constantly to keep the body in a state of equilibrium and health. Virtually every cell in your body has mechanisms that are activated in the presence of toxins to protect itself and its neighbours.

ONE MAN'S MEAT IS ANOTHER'S TOXIN

So what exactly are these toxins that the liver is detoxing us from? The answer to this might surprise many. In the words of the 16th-century Swiss physician Paracelsus, 'only the dose makes the poison.'[3] It is all about dose; most substances are fine in small amounts and almost everything becomes toxic at a high enough dose. What constitutes a high dose very much depends on what the compound is, and the person taking it. Medicines, for instance, are what most of us would think of immediately when we discuss dose. We all know that it is wise to take what the doctor tells you or what it says on the back of the pack; taking too much and overdosing on prescription drugs is simply not something most of us would intentionally do. Yet the same is true for nearly all substances, some with scary-sounding names, others seemingly benign. For example, metals like iron and magnesium are required by our bodies in small amounts, but rapidly become toxic at high levels. Whatever you may think of pesticides, the levels you might find on a (non-organic) vegetable or fruit or nut are highly unlikely to kill you. Yet, ingesting even a small amount of the undiluted pesticide probably would. Botulinum toxin, commercially known as botox, is a product of the bacteria *Clostridium botulinum* and is used (ill-advisedly I would suggest, although who am I to judge?) as a cosmetic tool by some to reduce the visible signs of wrinkles and 'crow's feet'. But get the dose even slightly wrong and it is one of the most dangerous toxins known to man.

The same, too, is true for all foods, including fruits and vegetables (before all of you begin throwing bananas at me, please hear me out). Carrots, for example, are clearly great for you, either raw or cooked or put in a soup, yet if you eat too many, like a bin bag's worth (highly unlikely for most people), you would get poisoned by the beta-carotene, which gives carrots their orange colour. This is a condition known as beta carotenemia, where you essentially end up with a carroty-orange tinge to your skin. This is not unique to carrots; too much (but, like, wayyyyy too much) squash, pumpkins, sweet potatoes and other orange-coloured produce would have the same effect. Another example is coconut water, which is refreshing and hydrating but has very high levels of potassium. There have been reported cases of people rushed to the hospital after suffering from fainting spells and abnormal heart rhythms due to hyperkalaemia (high blood potassium) from overdoing the coconut water. Higher potassium levels are also found in bananas and some vegetables, such as kale. Finally, broccoli and other members of the brassica family actually contain trace amounts of formaldehyde. So in principle, you could get formaldehyde poisoning by eating too much broccoli. Granted, you would have to eat a whole lot of bananas and drink quite a bit of coconut water or broccoli juice to end up being poisoned, but my point is that too much of a good thing, 'natural' or not, will eventually become a bad thing, a toxic thing.

IS 'NATURAL' SUGAR BETTER FOR YOU?

At this point, many of you might be thinking that juicing doesn't actually sound that bad. For one thing, fruit juices in particular taste fantastic; they are refreshing, sometimes they are zingy, they come in a huge assortment of colours and flavours, and all of them are sweet, which of course is what makes them taste fantastic. The one thing you get a lot of in fruit juices is sugar. There is nearly as much sugar in a glass of orange juice (8 grams/100 mls or 8 per cent) and apple juice (10 per cent) as there is in Coca-Cola (10.6 per cent). However, surely the fact that the sugar in juice is 'natural', coming as it has from fruit, means it is better for you then the refined stuff added to soda? Absolutely not true. The vast majority of sugar in juice and in soda is sucrose, which is a disaccharide formed of one molecule of glucose and one molecule of fructose. So sucrose, when broken down, becomes 50 per cent glucose and 50 per cent fructose. The sucrose added to soda might be refined, but it would have come from sugar cane or sugar beet, so is also 'natural'. How about sugar from honey or maple syrup or agave nectar? They are often marketed as better for you, or more curiously, as a 'sugar-free' alternative. (*Great British Bake Off* and your 'sugar-free' week, I'm looking at you.) This is just simply not true. They do of course taste different because one is in effect bee puke, another is tree sap and another concentrated cactus (well, not technically a cactus, but cactus-like) juice, so naturally each brings its own distinct flavour to different recipes. But they are sweet because of sugar.

In some countries, high-fructose corn syrup is used to sweeten sodas and baked goods instead. High-fructose corn syrup is made by enzymatically converting cornstarch (which would be mostly chains of glucose) to an approximately 50 per cent glucose and 50 per cent fructose mixture. Why not just use pure glucose? Because pure glucose, if you've ever tried it, tastes very odd and is almost unpalatable. The yummy flavour in sugar actually comes from the fructose portion. So in spite of the name, 'high'-fructose corn syrup contains about as much fructose as sucrose. Some people don't like the fact that corn syrup is the product of an industrial process, and we can certainly debate the pros and cons of the increasing use of such products. But the incontrovertible and unequivocal fact of the matter is that sugar is sugar, whatever its source, wherever it comes from.

IS SUGAR BAD FOR YOU?

This will probably be an unpopular response, but the answer is that it entirely depends on how much you consume. At the risk of sounding like a broken record, it is a question of dose. When you eat an apple or an orange, you are taking in sugar. However, it probably takes five or six oranges to make a glass of orange juice. Would you ever eat six oranges in one sitting? Very unlikely. Yet you would give almost no thought to consuming six oranges' worth of sugar in a single glass of juice during breakfast, which, as I pointed out above, is no different from the amount of sugar you'd get from drinking a soda at breakfast. Another problem is the delivery of sugar as a liquid. Sugar is calorically dense, and when you dissolve it into a liquid, you can suddenly deliver hundreds of calories into your system in literally seconds. When you eat anything, whether or not it is sweet, you have to first chew the food. As you do this, you begin to salivate, which your gastrointestinal tract senses, and as a result begins to prepare itself for nutrients to arrive, including secreting hormones and adjusting your metabolism. The hormones that are secreted when solid food is consumed are what make you eventually feel full and stop eating. When your calories are in the form of a sweet drink, however, they pass through the stomach, into the small intestine and are very rapidly absorbed with no digestion. As no digestion has occurred, the release of hormones that make you feel full is delayed, and as a result, you end up eating more than you actually required. If you like sweet things, it is far better to eat them than it is to drink them.

In addition to the release of hormones that will eventually make you feel full if you actually eat fruit, there is the important benefit of consuming the fibre found in the fruit. Fibre plays a crucial role in gut health, both for motility and to nourish your gut bacteria. Additionally, the fibre reduces the caloric availability of the sugar in the fruit, which means you also get less sugar. The vast majority of the fibre found in fruit and in vegetables is lost during the juicing process, whether or not you favour cold-press or use a centrifugal juicer.

CLEANSES DON'T CLEANSE

There are other 'cleanses' on the market aside from juicing. How about a veggie-smoothie cleanse, which would contain very little sugar, but would have fibre? Fibre and no sugar, surely that would be a great cleanse? There is a green-tea cleanse, which also doesn't contain sugar and instead has loads of antioxidants? How about the water fasting cleanse? Then there is the alkaline cleanse, which involves consuming raw, fresh, alkaline soups, juices and smoothies for a period of between three and ten days.

OK, please let me be clear. Some of the stuff in these cleanses is actually going to be good for you. Fruit juice is great for you in moderation and a veggie smoothie is even better. Others follow the 'dose makes the poison' rule. So, green tea, being as I am Chinese, is something that I have drunk since I was a little kid. It is a source of antioxidants, particularly the catechin epigallocatechin gallate (EGCG). But if you drink too much of it or, worse, if you take green-tea extract as a pill, you could take too much of the EGCG antioxidant and run the risk of damaging your liver.[4] The 'water fast' is just fasting . . . you'll just feel really awful and end up losing weight; and the alkaline approach is absolute nonsense (I discuss this in detail in the next chapter).

None of these, however, 'cleanse' you. They may supply nutrients, they may poison you, they may help you lose weight and they may do nothing at all. But the bottom line is, cleanses do not cleanse you. Your liver and kidneys 'cleanse' you.

WHEN YOUR LIVER IS NOT WORKING

As a brief aside, let's have a look at what happens when the liver isn't working optimally, as it really highlights its importance to our health. My dad, together with his inability to metabolise lactose, also cannot drink alcohol; like, literally a single drop. I remember on the day I graduated from university, our department hosted a champagne drinks reception for all of the proud parents. My proud dad took a glass, and all he did was sniff it, and the minute quantities of alcohol being aerosoled into my dad's nose by the bubbles was enough to make him turn pink! I took the glass away from him because he was on photography duty that day to capture me on stage in my big moment, years of hard work in the making. The reason for this is that he, like many other Chinese folk, have a deficiency in the enzymes that metabolise alcohol.[5] These enzymes, alcohol dehydrogenase and acetaldehyde dehydrogenase, are localised to the liver. After having a drink, the blood carrying alcohol is filtered through the liver, where, if the enzymes are working, alcohol is then metabolised. If however, like in my dad, they are not, then the alcohol, even minute amounts of it, continues to circulate in the blood for a long time, so he can end up being quite tipsy on even the smallest quantities of bubbly wine.

Then there are situations where your liver is actually physically damaged. Your liver plays a key role in metabolising lipids. However, when you have a number of highly fatty meals in a row, lipids can end up accumulating in your liver cells, resulting in a 'fatty liver'. This is exactly what happens in *foie gras*, when the liver of a duck or goose is fattened by force-feeding it corn. *Foie gras* literally means 'fat liver' in French. Normally, your fatty liver is reversible with a change in diet, but it does kinda put me off my food, albeit fleetingly, if I think too hard about my liver turning from deep purple to light pink as it fills up with fat. The problems begin when your liver stays fatty for too long. In those who are susceptible (around 40 per cent of people with fatty liver), this long-term and large increase of fat in the liver, which is not its natural state, causes damage and is accompanied by inflammation. This results in a situation referred to as 'steatohepatitis' or fatty liver disease.[6] At its most severe, this steatohepatitis can lead to 'liver cirrhosis', which is scarring that occurs in response to damage to the liver. Each time the liver is injured, it tries to repair itself, and in the process, scar tissue forms. As more and more scar tissue forms, it makes it difficult for the liver to function.

Another way of getting fatty liver disease is through alcohol abuse. What does alcohol have to do with a fatty liver, you might ask? Well, the liver is where alcohol is metabolised; as a consequence, abuse of alcohol, which is also not a natural state, will eventually damage the liver. Because another key role of the liver is lipid metabolism, if your liver is irreparably damaged by alcohol, it is then unable to metabolise lipids effectively, resulting in accumulation of lipids, fatty liver disease, leading, in some, to liver cirrhosis. Two different causes of liver damage, but with the same result.

A little-known fact is that sugar can also play a role in the health or not of the liver.[7] Sucrose, as I mentioned, is broken down to glucose and fructose. As long as you are not diabetic, glucose is almost immediately taken up by your skeletal muscles and your fat after a meal, in response to insulin. Fructose, however, ends up in the liver, where, if not used immediately, it is actually converted to fat. So if you are knocking back serious amounts of sugar, which is what you would effectively be doing during a 'fruit juice cleanse', you are actually putting your liver under pressure. Ironic, given that one of the juice cleanse claims is that it is giving your liver a break. Nothing could be further from the truth.

One of the overt signs that all is not right with the liver is jaundice, which many of us would recognise as a yellowing of the skin and eyes. When red blood cells have completed their life span of approximately 120 days, they have to be broken down and excreted, and this is one of the primary roles of the liver. The oxygen-carrying component of red blood cells is called haemoglobin, which is also what gives the cells, and hence blood, its deep red colour. One of the breakdown products of haemoglobin is 'bilirubin', which is yellowish in colour and becomes a key part of bile, which is produced by the liver and secreted into the small intestine where it aids the digestion of lipids. Some bilirubin is also excreted via urine. In fact, bilirubin is actually what gives faeces and urine their distinct colour. When the liver is not working however, instead of being shunted to bile, the yellow bilirubin stays in the circulation, resulting in jaundice. Jaundice is therefore not a disease *per se*, but a symptom of a liver that is not working well.

In fact, with over 500 known functions, the role of the liver is nigh-on impossible to replicate. For instance, while you can undergo kidney dialysis when your kidney fails, there is, certainly at the time of writing, no 'liver-dialysis' procedure yet available. While the liver is famously able to regenerate, it can only do so from regions that are not cirrhotic, so when too much cirrhosis has occurred, the liver then begins to fail. There is currently no way to compensate for the absence of liver function in the long term. When this happens, the only option remaining is a liver transplant. Liver failure is, tragically, incompatible with life.

So I guess the message is, rather than going on detoxes and cleanses, the best thing you can do is to look after your liver.

RAW FOOD DETOX

I was on the train heading from Cambridge to London recently, when I met an owner of a 'raw-food' business (isn't that just the vegetable counter at the supermarket?), who tried to explain to me her 'raw' philosophy.

'If you leave a raw onion in the shed or put it into the ground, it will grow. Whereas when you do the same with a cooked onion, it will rot. Do you see what I mean?'

Ummmm, no? Did she think that cooked food would rot us? I'm not sure she knew what she meant.

Raw foodies define 'raw food' as anything that has not been refined, canned or chemically processed, and has not been heated above 48°C (118°F). They claim that heating your food above 48°C destroys some of the natural enzymes in food, so the body overworks itself by having to produce more of its own enzymes, exhausting its energy; explaining the raw onion story above. Wow, there is just so much to pick apart in this claim. Cooking your food will not only destroy some of the natural enzymes, it will destroy pretty much all of the enzymes in the food. Crucially, however, so will the acid in your stomach. Whatever hardy enzymes and other proteins that do survive that acidic cauldron of the stomach will then be fully digested in the small intestines before being absorbed into our system. When we consume another organism, everything is broken down into their basic building blocks, and reassembled in each cell according to the instructions on our own human DNA. Most of us, I hope, understand that if you eat an antelope, it won't make us run faster, nor would having a kangaroo steak make you jump any higher. Likewise, we do not eat beef or salmon or for that matter broccoli that has not been heated above 48°C, and are then able to co-opt their enzymes whole, to use in our own bodies. That is simply not how biology works. Cooking in fact actually saves our body energy, while increasing the caloric availability of food!

Another claim is that if you cook your food above 57°C (134°F; these are some very specific temperatures), it destroys heat-sensitive nutrients. This is of course true; the classic example being vitamin C, which is famously heat sensitive. We get around that by eating much of our fruit, and some of our vegetables, which are of course rich in vitamin C, raw. This is undoubtedly something we don't do enough of and is to be encouraged. Equally, however, cooking many other foods makes nutrients more available to us. For example, cooking carrots and tomatoes makes it easier for our bodies to benefit from their protective antioxidants, and cooking sweetcorn allows us to access the niacin more easily. The challenge for anyone on a raw-food diet is getting enough protein, vitamin B12 and iron, as these nutrients are typically found in foods that are best heated above 57°C, including meat, fish, eggs and grains. Cooking, of course, also kills most parasites that might be present in the food, which surely is a good thing . . . otherwise you might end up losing weight for entirely the wrong reason!

IS IT A BIRD, IS IT A PLANE, IS IT A SUPERFOOD?

As a complement to cleanses, and detoxes, I can't not touch on superfoods before leaving this chapter. Goji berries, blueberries, kale, avocado, wheatgrass, cinnamon, quinoa and garlic. Aside from being members of the plant kingdom, what do all of these foods have in common? They have achieved the status of 'superfoods'. These foods are of course all good for you, containing vitamins, minerals and fibre; some, like cinnamon, may very well have medicinal qualities, and garlic has the added advantage of being able to repel vampires. But are they 'super' in any way?

Since the beginning of humankind, eating some foods has been thought to slow down ageing, or lift depression, or boost our physical ability, make us cleverer, heal us and stop pain. Some of these, such as the extract of willow leaves used to relieve pain and lower fevers, genuinely do work, as the chemical salicylate found in the extract is a precursor to aspirin. Others, however, are simply old-wives' tales or witch doctors' cures with no evidence of being effective at all. To my mind, superfoods are the modern equivalent, each having some supposed magical health property, with many of us, for instance, desperate to believe that eating a single fruit or vegetable containing a certain antioxidant will zap a diseased or cancerous cell. While the superfoods I have listed (and there are many more available that I haven't listed here) are indeed healthy, and each contains some genuinely important nutrients (antioxidants in berries) or healthy fats (avocados), these days eating enough is suddenly not enough. Eating MORE is better than eating enough. If something is good for you, surely more of a good thing is better?

Not true.

As I've said already, there is a healthy and a toxic dose for most foods. Remember, *only the dose makes the poison*.

CLEANSE AND DETOX? GIVE IT A BREAK

I had the most fascinating conversation with Sarah that first day we met, and happily, she ended up helping me research the chapter you are reading now, as well as Chapters 4 and 10, for which I will always be grateful.

The bottom line is, there is currently no scientific evidence to support the supposed benefits of juice cleansing or of detox. The marketing of this sector plays into the misconception that cleansing and detoxing are vital to the maintenance of bodily functions, therefore it would be in our best interest to undertake one or we risk developing chronic and terminal illnesses. The truth is, none of the purveyors of 'detox' products can tell you what we are supposed to be detoxing from, let alone show that using their product will reduce said unknown, yet potentially deadly, toxin. To rid ourselves of toxins, we simply need to have a well-functioning liver that you can achieve by eating sensibly and limiting consumption of substances, such as alcohol or large amounts of fructose, which cause it to work harder. Excessive consumption of any food can and will contribute to an increased load on the liver.

Juice cleanses are being sold as a philosophy of life; those that undertake them will emerge cleaner, more balanced, free of stress – ultimately a better version of themselves, superior to both their previous selves and uncleansed counterparts. This idea is not new. Cleansing or fasting practices are found in every major religion, to purify both body and soul. Generally speaking, however, for most people, detox and cleanse are typically confined to the month of January, and tends to mean drinking a little less, eating more healthily and getting a reasonable amount of exercise. Of course you will feel better! But you do not need any special products and you do not need to spend any money to do this. The evidence-backed approach, boring though it is, is that a healthy, well-balanced diet based on national guidelines is still the best 'cleanse and detox' available.

CHAPTER 9

The alkaline swindle

The first day of filming for the BBC's *Clean Eating* investigative programme was remarkable to me for a number of reasons. First of all, as we were in California it felt almost like a homecoming of sorts. Well, we were in San Diego, which is more than 500 miles south of San Francisco ... but at least I was in the same time-zone. Second, I got to drive that Ford Mustang convertible for the first time in my life! I know, I know, boys and their toys, how very clichéd. Third, and most remarkable of all, was my surreal visit and interview with Robert Young at his pH Miracle Ranch.

Robert Young's pH Miracle Ranch, also called the *Rancho del Sol* (The Sun Ranch), is an avocado and grapefruit ranch in Valley Center, North San Diego County, California. It is named after, and paid for by, his 'pH Miracle' series of books, of which Robert claims

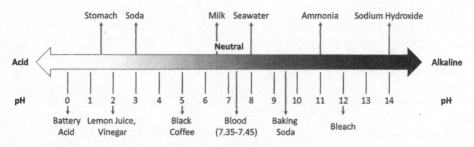

FIGURE 9 pH values of key substances

to have sold more than four million copies. Robert's central thesis is that '*the single measurement most important to your health is the pH of your blood and tissues – how acid or alkaline it is*',[1] and he believes that in order to maintain this perfect state of health, we have to eat 'alkaline' foods and avoid 'acidic' foods.

This is a story of that visit.

ALKALINITY AND ACIDITY

Just a very quick reminder to all of us who have forgotten most of our high-school chemistry: pH is a measure of the concentration of hydrogen ions (H^+) in a solution; 'p' coming from the German *potenz*, meaning power or concentration, and the 'H' for hydrogen. The pH scale goes from 0 to 14, indicating how acidic or alkaline a solution is. The middle of the scale is 7, which is neutral. Any number below that is acidic and any number above 7 is alkaline. The scale is 'logarithmic', meaning that it jumps by factors of ten. So a substance with a pH 5 is ten times more acidic than a pH 6 substance and pH 4 is ten times more acidic than pH 5; while on the other side of neutral, a pH of 9 is ten times more alkaline than pH 8, and pH 10 ten times more alkaline than pH 9. So in reality, it takes quite a lot to shift the pH of a particular solution. The figure opposite shows the pH of some relevant solutions and substances.

Typical highly acidic substances are lemon juice, vinegar, our own stomach acid and battery acid. The highly alkaline end includes ammonia, bleach and sodium hydroxide, which are very caustic and thus often used as cleaning solutions. Black coffee and milk are slightly acidic; and blood, at pH 7.35-7.45, is indeed slightly alkaline, so Robert is at least partially correct in thinking of humans as alkaline beings.

THE PH MIRACLE

As I entered the house, Robert showed me around, past the empty spherical fish tank built into the wall on one side of the living area, and then into the kitchen, where he was keen I share his daily routine. Robert proceeded to thrust a large glass of dark green juice my way. I looked suspiciously at it and gave it a sniff, cognisant that being violently ill at the beginning of a visit was, ideally, not quite the polite thing to do.

'Is this sweet or savoury?' I asked Robert.

Instead of answering my question, Robert said 'It's wheatgrass . . . Look, I'll join you.' He had, sitting on the kitchen counter, one of these plastic water-bottles with a giant straw sticking out the top, that was filled to the brim with this green juice, from which he took an impressively large gulp. Robert didn't go green and in fact looked like he was enjoying the drink, so I took a tentative sip . . . and it turned out tasting like cold green tea. It was, as it turned out, quite pleasant.

Robert was about my height, had pale hair, almost bleached (I'm no expert but it looked to me like it was natural); and he had a trimmed moustache and goatee combo that was darker than his hair. He carried more weight around his middle than was healthy, but then again he was in his mid-sixties when I interviewed him, and given my own wobbly middle, I certainly shouldn't be throwing any stones! Robert's original *pH Miracle* book, which he wrote with his wife Shelly, was published in 2002.

'I think I read somewhere . . . you call yourself a "world renowned" microbiologist?'

These were actually Robert's own words that I had read, right at the front of *The pH Miracle*.[2]

'I don't know that you need to put "world renowned" in front of it . . .'

Robert claims a passion for biology, particularly the field of hae-matology, which is the study of blood. Robert's interest in blood primarily revolves around its pH. Robert's theory, which I want to stress was developed outside of the mainstream and at the edges of academic credibility, was that certain foods caused acid to build up in the body. If there was too much acid, then it couldn't be balanced by the blood, and this acid ends up in our tissues. Robert believes that pH imbalance in our blood leads to signs of disease such as, 'low energy, fatigue, poor digestion ... foggy thinking, aches and pains, as well as major disorders.'[3] He also argues that overacidity is what's keeping (us) fat.'[4] In contrast, maintaining the pH balance of blood is key to our health, leading to 'energy, mental clarity, smooth operation of all body systems, clear, bright eyes and skin, and a lean, trim body.'[5] He claims that with the programme in *The pH Miracle*, all this will be yours within weeks.

Clear bright eyes? What are we, Labradors? Trout?

THE ALKALINE DIET

Robert and I walked out of the kitchen and on to the patio out back, where there was a large swimming pool and, beyond that, a seating area with sun umbrellas and patio heaters. It was a warm and sunny day, and the whole scene could not have been more Californian if it had tried. It was heavenly. (As I am writing this exact sentence, I am sitting at my desk in Cambridge, looking out the window to a cold and dreary January morning ... I love it here really, but boy, do January and February days get me wishing for the sun, the sand and the sea.) When we walked past the pool, it was clear that the main residence of the pH Miracle Ranch was perched on the side of a hill. The ranch stretched for 46 acres down the hill and was covered in avocado trees. Robert pointed to the hills beyond and told me that Steve Jobs used to own an estate there. I did not fact-check that. As we walked along a land-scaped path taking us down the hill, we passed gardeners pruning trees.

'We're right now cutting back the avocado trees. Avocado is what I refer to as God's butter. So possibly the perfect food.'

According to Robert, *The pH Miracle* programme was very simple. Eighty per cent of one's diet must be composed of 'alkalising' foods, leaving 20 per cent for 'acid' foods. The trick, of course, is to know what foods are alkalising and what foods are acidic. Helpfully, Robert has produced colourful and detailed charts. I won't, however, reproduce any of these charts here for two key reasons.

First, while many of the charts attributed to *The pH Miracle* include a pH scale of sorts, going from 0 to 14, what Robert has designated as acid or alkalising has little to do with the actual pH of those foods. For example, he lists lemons and limes as alkalising, and thus good for you and should form part of the 80 per cent. I have no doubt that lemons and limes, packed as they are with vitamin C and other nutrient goodies, are fabulous for one's diet. The problem is that vitamin C is known as ascorbic *acid*, and lemons and limes also contain citric *acid* (they are citrus fruits after all). As a result, lemon juice actually has a very acidic pH of 2. He lists all meat as being acidic, except for the inconvenient truth that meat contains blood, which is, as we have established, slightly alkaline. There are also examples of foods, which, according to Robert, change pH when heated. Robert argues that most foods get more acidic when cooked. Now, vitamin C is heat sensitive and tends to get destroyed in the cooking process. But that would mean, if anything, that citrus fruits become *less* acidic when cooked. He says that raw unpasteurised milk is neutral in pH, but becomes acidic when pasteurised. Milk is indeed slightly acidic with a pH of 6.5. But that is its pH whether or not it has been through the pasteurisation process, it doesn't change. In fact, because pasteurisation reduces the number of living bacteria in milk, it slows down the fermentation process, which produces lactic acid. Then there are foods that appear to vary in their pH depending on their domestication status. For instance, 'wild' rice, which I take to mean is rice that comes in a variety of colours, is alkalising, whereas brown rice and white 'polished' rice are both considered acidic. These are just a few of the more egregious examples. But in essence, I can see no scientific rhyme or reason for what foods Robert lists as acid or alkali.

Second, even if you could bring yourself to accept Robert's food taxonomy, it completely ignores the presence of our stomach, which at pH 1.5 is, by quite a long way, the most acidic compartment in our body. Thus, everything we eat, whether lemons, meat or avocados (God's alkaline butter), becomes acidified by the stomach before it passes into the small intestine. I brought this fact up with Robert. His response, delivered with breathtaking confidence, was that the stomach was not actually acidic at all. It was the stomach's job to extract acid from food as it passes through to the small intestine, which is the only reason it was acidic.

I was, in an extremely unusual occurrence, at a loss for words.

OUR BLOOD IS AT AN ALKALINE PH

Just so there is absolutely no room for doubt, the stomach juices are demonstrably and unequivocally acidic. The bottom line is, there is NO evidence, none whatsoever, that your blood's pH can be influenced by what you eat. The pH of our blood is very tightly regulated, sitting as it does between pH 7.35 – 7.45; not by our diet, but by our kidneys and lungs through homeostasis. Homeostasis is the ability of the body to maintain stability within its internal environment when dealing with external changes. It controls much of our physiological processes, including, for example, our body temperature, our thirst, our hunger, our blood sugar levels, our blood pressure and our blood pH.

There is an easy way of raising the pH of your blood, and that is through hyperventilation. Carbon dioxide, when dissolved in a liquid, is acidic. The slightly alkaline pH of our blood is the result of, amongst many other factors, a carefully controlled concentration of carbon dioxide. When you hyperventilate or over-breathe, you eliminate more carbon dioxide from the blood than your body is producing, which results in your blood pH going UP; i.e. becoming more alkaline. Your body should normally attempt to compensate for this. If it fails, however, you end up with 'respiratory alkalosis', which include symptoms of dizziness, tingling in the lips, hands or feet, headache, weakness, fainting and seizures. Please don't try hyperventilating at home.

On the other side of the pH scale is diabetic ketoacidosis. Type 1 diabetes is an autoimmune condition where insulin-producing cells in the pancreas have been destroyed. Normally of course, type 1 diabetics are treated with regular injections of insulin, so that their blood glucose levels are controlled. In untreated or poorly controlled type 1 diabetes, however, because your muscles and fat are unable to absorb any glucose, you would end up burning only fat, producing uncontrolled amounts of ketones. Because ketone bodies are acidic, a large accumulation would dangerously lower the pH of the blood, thus the name ketoacidosis, which if left unchecked can be fatal.

The bottom line is, in extreme cases when homeostasis fails, and your blood pH goes measurably above 7.45, such as in respiratory alkalosis, or below 7.35, such as in ketoacidosis, you will know about it. And if you don't do anything about it pretty quickly, usually involving a trip to a hospital emergency room, you will likely end up dead. I think we can all agree that this could ruin your weekend and is probably best avoided.

SUPPLEMENTS TO HELP ACHIEVE PH BALANCE?

In addition to eating the alkaline way, Robert also recommends 'high-quality' supplements that help achieve and maintain pH balance. There are simply too many for me to list here, but here are the 'stars', which he recommends you should take every day:

a) **Hydrogen-peroxide drops**, which you should put into your water and drink at least four litres a day. It apparently alkalises the water and also releases O_2 to help kill terrible acid bugs. (Please don't, under any circumstances, drink hydrogen peroxide; people use it to clean the wax out of ears, and it will result in an extremely unpleasant death if you get the dose wrong.)

b) **Concentrated green powder from plants**. This will largely be chlorophyll, which are the tiny organelles in plants that perform photosynthesis and is primarily what gives plants their green colouration. You apparently add a teaspoon of this stuff to your hydrogen, peroxide, treated water in order to gently pull your blood and tissues from acidic to alkaline, so as to help achieve an ideal pH balance. At the very least, this explains my wheatgrass juice experience. Wait, was there hydrogen peroxide in that drink?! Ack! Ack!

c) **Multivitamin pills**. Vitamins are nutrients that act as co-factors for a number of essential enzymes, and are therefore required for the normal functioning of our body. Robert argues that our modern environment, from the way food is grown to the way it is cooked and processed, has destroyed much of the endogenous vitamin content. This is simply not true. Discussing vitamin supplements in any useful manner would require a whole other book of its own. Suffice to say, while we all need a certain amount of vitamins, taking more than you need has no additional benefits, and in some circumstances can actually be harmful.

d) **Essential fatty acids, such as omega 3 and 6**. This is the one supplement I don't have a problem with; although in reality if you eat enough oily fish and olive oil, you shouldn't need more.

Incidentally, all of these supplements, and more, are available for sale on Robert's website; all major credit cards accepted. A quarter pound (113 grams) of 'green powder', for example, will set you back nearly USD$40. Gosh, living the healthy and alkaline way certainly doesn't come cheap.

PH INFLUENCE

At this point, we sat down to an alkaline lunch, prepared by Robert's cook. We were joined by a colleague of Robert's, a lady with long dark-brown hair, possibly in her mid-fifties, who was an expert at scanning your body to find patches of 'acidity'. She did offer to scan me, but I politely turned down the offer. I didn't want to have any of my unsuspecting 'acid patches' displayed on national TV, thank you. The director and crew cried off joining us for lunch, saying they had to work; they had to film the event after all. Cowards.

Lunch was, as it happened, very good. We had a very tasty vegan and gluten-free minestrone soup to start, a kale salad with a lovely sesame seed and olive oil dressing, and a gluten-free vegetable wrap with an avocado sauce (it tasted very much like guacamole but had the consistency of a thick soup). An alkaline diet essentially consists of vegetables, many of them raw, with little to no meat. It is gluten-free, and aside from wild rice and a few other oddities, is nearly grain-free and very low in carbohydrates. It also strongly discourages refined sugars and alcohol; and aside from olive oil, is very low in fat. As a result, the alkaline diet is undoubtedly very healthy. While it is not as extreme as a plant-based diet (hooray for avocados and olive oil), it is certainly not a million miles away, and is still very restrictive in what you can eat. What this means is that many people do end up losing quite substantial amounts of weight while following an alkaline diet. As we have discussed in previous chapters, weight loss is the most effective way to reduce your risk for a number of different diseases, so is always a very useful aim. The alkaline diet, however, is quite a complex diet, in that it is mired in obscure rules. Whatever you might think of 'grain-free', 'gluten-free' or 'plant-based' diets, at least their names are actually descriptive of the diet. There is however, no way of deciphering an alkaline diet from first principles, because it is not based on any principles that you or I would understand. You have to buy *The pH Miracle*, you have to refer to one of Robert's many colourful charts.

Yet, in spite of its pseudoscientific complexity, the alkaline diet has had tremendous reach and influence, even extending to two key characters that we have already met in earlier chapters. For example, Bill Davis has an entire chapter in *Wheat Belly* (Chapter 8) that is entitled 'Dropping acid: Wheat as the great pH disruptor'.[6] Robert Young does indeed view wheat through an acidic lens. While in Chapter 10 of *The China Study*, Colin Campbell argues that 'animal protein, unlike plant protein, increases the acid load in the body. An increased acid load means that our blood and tissues become more acidic',[7] which is, of course, consistent with Robert's view. However, given that Bill advocates meat in a big way, who are we, the unsuspecting public, supposed to believe? Dr Davis? Prof Campbell? 'Dr' Young?

In the UK, one of the key promoters of the alkaline diet is Honestly Healthy, the health-food brand created by the duo Natasha Corrett and Vicki Edgson. In talking about one of their books, *Honestly Healthy Cleanse*, Natasha Corrett says about Robert Young:

'*Unfortunately, his work . . . isn't recognised by the medical industry, perhaps because giant pharmaceutical organisations wouldn't be able to make money out of doctors prescribing vegetables.*'[8]

Here we go again, yet another 'health-food aficionado' sticking the knife into 'big pharma'. I was curious to hear from Robert about the spread and influence of alkaline living, and had brought along, more as a prop than anything, the health-food duo's first book, *Honestly Healthy: Eat with your body in mind, the alkaline way*. I asked him if he knew of the people behind the brand, Natasha Corrett and Vicki Edgson.

'Yes. Two of my students who have been studying my work for years. They actually called me when they were producing this book because they wanted my impressions on it.'[9]

Whoa, hold up there. That answer took me entirely by surprise . . . it certainly didn't come up in any of our research preparing for this interview. The manner with which he responded indicated to me that there was at least some truth to the statement. Director Tristan Quinn did not react, and Cameraman Kevin White and soundman Ali Pares coolly kept the camera and sound recording. I continued innocently.

'So you saw a draft?'

'Yeah, I saw a draft of the book. So I'm happy to help anyone that is interested in helping others feel better, look better and live a better life and it comes right down to food.'

When we got back to the UK, we spoke to the book's publisher, who told us they never consulted Robert directly or sent him proofs. We reached out to Natasha, but she declined our invite to be interviewed on the programme. She later explained in a post on her Instagram account that she turned down our invite because 'I wanted to have a chance to put my view across without it being edited in a way that could be misinterpreted or spun by anyone like before.'[10]

Sticks and stones, Natasha, sticks and stones.

In that same Instagram post, Natasha denied Robert's claim that both she and Vicki were students of his, or that she had sent him proofs of their first book, and to be clear, there was no reason for me not to believe her. Natasha also said that 'by no means is his [Robert's] plan a basis for our brand'. However, '... the alkaline way' does appear in the title of Honestly Healthy's first book and the Amazon website calls it 'the original alkaline diet cookbook'.[11] They also put little pink hearts on each of their recipes to indicate the level of alkalinity; the scale goes from one to three hearts with increasing alkalinity, depending on the types of ingredients used.[12] The basis for this cutesy heart scale is the acid/alkaline food taxonomy set out by Robert in *The pH Miracle*, including considering lemons as 'alkaline'.

PLEOMORPHISM

Robert Young's view that alkalinity is good and acidity is bad goes beyond food.

'All sickness and disease can be prevented by managing the delicate pH balance of the fluids of the body'.

Robert has based much of the 'science' of alkaline living on Antoine Béchamp's microzymian theory.[13] Pierre Jacques Antoine Béchamp (1816–1908) was a French scientist who did not believe in cells as the basic units of life, or that bacteria were one of the causes of infection and disease. Rather, Béchamp claimed that 'molecular granules', which he called microzymas, in biological fluids such as blood, were actually the basic units of life. In 'favourable' conditions, these microzymas would be turned into cells; however, in unfavourable host and environmental conditions, the microzymas would turn into bacteria and other microorganisms, resulting in disease. Béchamp called the process by which microzymas changed from one form to another, 'pleomorphism'; essentially a form of spontaneous generation. Béchamp's bitter rival at the time was Louis Pasteur (1822–95). Pasteur is regarded as the father of 'germ theory', that infection came from the outside. While he didn't originally propose it, he performed the experiments showing that without contamination, microorganisms could not develop. Pasteur demonstrated that in sterilised and sealed flasks nothing would grow, whereas if he sterilised a flask and then left it open, bacteria and other microorganisms would rapidly grow, and in doing so proved that 'germ theory' was correct. He then went on to develop the principles of vaccination, microorganism-based fermentation and pasteurisation, which was only possible with the understanding of germ theory. In doing so, Pasteur comprehensively disproved Béchamp's microzymian theory of pleomorphism.[14] Yet today, Béchamp's work continues to be promoted by a small group of germ-theory denialists (yes, they are a thing) and alternative-medicine proponents. They claimed that mainstream science of the time, led by Pasteur, waged a campaign to silence Béchamp, which is why germ theory predominates today. Included amongst these denialists is Robert Young.

Robert believes that under healthy alkaline conditions, the microzymas in the blood exist largely as blood cells. When one is eating acidic foods, however, the blood undergoes pleomorphism, and transforms into disease-causing bacteria. Robert claimed to have seen this happening in real-time, using 'live blood analysis', which was, as far as I could gather, putting a drop of blood onto a slide, and analysing it by staring at it down a microscope. Robert had actually posted a video online of 'live blood analysis' of a type 1 diabetic patient. He claimed it showed a red blood cell transforming into bacteria. I have had a look at the video and what I saw were unidentified cells, and something moving amongst them. I speak as someone who uses microscopes for research purposes. Typically, in order to tell what cells we are looking at, you would need to mark them somehow. Different cells will have different proteins on their surface, and you can target fluorescent anti-bodies that emit a known colour to those proteins. So you might, for instance, be able to distinguish different types of neurons, or neurons from non-neurons, or even see an infection by yeast or bacteria. Robert's video provided no such marks, so there was no way to tell whether what we were looking at was blood, let alone if a blood cell was undergoing pleomorphism. Crucially, none of this of course was scientifically plausible.

When I posed this to him, he called it 'the new biology'; he said it was 'a new thought, a new consideration'. He talks about this 'new biology' consistently throughout *The pH Miracle*. These thoughts were, by definition of course, not 'new', based as they were on Béchamp's thoroughly disproven 19th-century theory. In reality, these were just his fantasy. It was 'post-truth'.

AN ADJECTIVE AND NOT A NOUN

The problem was that for Robert, clinging on to this debunked theory was far more than an academic exercise, far more than just some other kooky diet. He believed that he was on to something; he believed he could cure, nay, reverse disease.

'Because disease is an illusion! In reality, what we call disease is the manifestation of the body struggling to prevent over-acidification ... of the body's cells, tissues, organs or glands. Disease is the body in preservation mode straining to maintain the homeostasis of its internal, alkaline fluids.'

Since Robert believed that all diseases were just a reflection of the spectrum of acidity in the body, if you follow his argument *ad absurdum*, then all diseases should be cured by the reversal of the acidity. This was where things shifted from eating avocados to something entirely darker. He began to believe that he could reverse cancer; that's right, the big 'C'. Below is an extended quote that I have taken from the 'introducing cancer' page of Robert's 'pHmiracleliving' website. Google it, I am not making any of this up.

'Cancer is the body in preservation mode trying to maintain its natural healthy alkaline design. So first, you must understand that cancer is unequivocally not a disease, but a symptom . . . All conditions of cancer potentially can be reversed if the treatments are focused on the fluids and not the cells of the body. Therefore it doesn't matter what the cancerous condition is, because cancer is not the cause but the effect of an over-acidic lifestyle and diet which is the cause of cancer.'[15]

Robert told me that he considered the word 'cancer' to be an adjective and not a noun; in other words, that it described the environment that enabled the disease, rather than the disease itself. Many of you reading this book will have been touched by cancer before, either directly or indirectly, and will find Robert's view of cancer shocking, possibly even offensive, running, as it does, completely at odds to the medical consensus.

Where does Robert's acidic view of cancer come from?

THE WARBURG EFFECT

Under healthy and normal conditions, an organ or tissue will stop growing once it reaches the appropriate size and shape. For instance, your kidney is kidney-shaped, each of the 206 bones in the adult human body have their own distinct shape but are yet comparable across all humans, and your stomach and intestine might be elastic, but still look like a stomach and intestine. Damaged cells might be replaced, but essentially once you become an adult, many of your organs will stay the same size and shape. What happens in malignant cancer, is that some of the cells lose their kidney or bone or stomach identity, and begin to replicate uncontrollably.

This resulting tumour, if not stopped and removed, will often end up killing the patient. Cancer cells, no matter their origin, tend to grow and replicate very quickly and thus have a higher metabolism than the surrounding normal tissue. As a result, they take up and use a lot of glucose. In normal tissue, glucose is combined with oxygen within our mitochondria, the power packs of our cells, and converted into energy, in a process known as oxidative phosphorylation. In cancer cells, one of the results of utilising so much glucose is that some of the glucose is converted into lactic *acid*, in a process called glycolysis. This increased use of glucose and the subsequent production of lactic acid is known as the Warburg effect,[16] named after Otto Warburg who made the original observations back in the 1920s. Thus, it is actually true that most cancers are acidic. Robert, once again, begins with a kernel of truth. However, where Robert gets it terribly wrong is that the lactic acid is not *causing* the cancer, it is being *produced* by the cancer. You can try and neutralise as much of the lactic acid coming from a cancer as possible, but that only removes one of the symptoms of cancer, it won't actually stop the cancer.

THE FALL OF YOUNG

A large part of the pH Miracle ranch had been set aside as a 'clinic' to treat cancer. To the right-hand side of the main residence was a small road, which if you followed it upwards, led to a number of small bungalows, a treatment facility and even a tennis court. It was here that Robert brought terminally ill patients to stay at his ranch for months at a time. During their stay, he would 'educate' them about the alkaline diet and lifestyle, provide massages, and then either infuse them intravenously with an alkaline solution, or use the solution as an enema. This solution was made using sodium bicarbonate, otherwise known as baking soda, which has a pH of 9.5; it is the same 'Arm and Hammer' stuff you stick into your fridge to absorb smells. Nope, I am not kidding. He convinced himself and he convinced his 'patients' that the sodium bicarbonate would reverse the acidity of cancer, and in turn reverse the cancer.

Please, under no circumstances should you infuse yourself with baking soda, nor should you stick it into your 'food to poop tube', from either end. Should you mess up the concentrations, you would kill yourself.

When I asked Robert how many cancer patients he had brought in for therapy, he didn't answer the question, but rather he said that he didn't treat cancer, but only educated and helped people understand lifestyle and diet.

In 2011, unsurprisingly but not soon enough, Robert's activities at the ranch attracted the attention of the Medical Board of California, which began an undercover investigation. They eventually gathered enough evidence to charge Robert. The district attorney's office told us that when they searched the ranch, they recovered 351 files relating to patients, although not all were cancer patients. People, as it turned out, went to see Robert for all sorts of issues: diabetes, lupus, weight loss, seizures, autism as well as digestive problems. Investigators established that at least 81 of the 351 patients treated at the ranch since 2005 were suffering from cancer. None of the 15 whose prognosis could be documented outlived it. One patient, Genia, died from congestive heart failure – fluid around the heart – while being treated.[17] As we toured the treatment facility, Robert showed us around one of the small bungalows where his patients would stay. We stepped into one of the bungalows as we were speaking of Genia.

'Where did she die?'

'Er, she died here.'

'In this room?!'

'That's what I understand, yes'

This was the second moment in the day that took me and the crew entirely by surprise. As before, camera and sound continued rolling unabated.

'She died here in this room?'

'Yes that's what I believe, yeah – I wasn't here – I was out of town.'

It was a sweltering day with temperatures in the mid-30s and the air-conditioner in the room was turned off; yet I felt a chill run down my spine. An invoice, which we obtained, documented thirty-three intravenous sodium-bicarbonate drips, each charged at USD$550, over thirty-one days; some administered by Robert himself. The cost of the IVs alone was north of USD$18,000.

'Who's given thirty IVs over thirty days?'

'They do that in hospitals through hydration but I'm not the doctor so I was not giving those IVs.'

'So you're washing your hands of all responsibility? Because you own the land – you own this space – this is your facility . . . '

'I'm not taking – no, it's not that I'm not taking responsibility that's why I'm in court and that's why I have this litigation, but no, I'm not – I am taking responsibility, you know, but the bottom line is, is that I ran a facility, er, for people to come, at their choosing, for a self-care programme.'

A self-care programme. I don't know about you, but I would have thought that any programme which required someone else to stick a needle into your arm and run an IV would disqualify itself to be described as 'self-care'.

Robert was convicted of two charges of practising medicine without a license, and was sentenced to three years and eight months in custody.[18] As part of the sentence, Robert had to make a public admission declaring that he was not a microbiologist, haematologist, medical or naturopathic doctor or trained scientist. However, good behaviour will cut that custodial sentence in half, and he was also credited for spending a year under house arrest.

So in reality, Robert will end up spending only about five months behind bars. By the time this book is out, Robert will once again be a free man.

THE ALKALINE SWINDLE

It was only the end of the first day of filming, and yet it had felt like a week; such were the revelations and range of emotions. Hellhole Canyon is a 1,907-acre nature reserve within a short drive of the pH Miracle Ranch. As we left the ranch after a surreal and shocking day, the crew and I stopped at a lookout point over the canyon to enjoy the beautiful sunset, the high clouds catching the colour, orange turning dark pink, and then slowly into dusk. It seemed an apt place to reflect on Robert Young's alkaline swindle. On the face of it, an alkaline diet, which encourages the consumption of lots of vegetables with little to no meat, is undoubtedly very healthy. The problem, however, is that it is sold not as a largely vegetarian diet, but as a pseudoscientific movement based on a questionable food pH scale, where citrus fruits are considered alkaline when they are clearly acidic, and meat acidic when it is demonstrably alkaline. So where is the harm, as long as it encourages the consumption of more veggies? First of all, if there are actually biologically plausible reasons why eating more vegetables is good for us, why invoke some convoluted other explanation instead? The whole thing, to be frank, reeks of some cynical marketing ploy, designed to carve out a lucrative niche in a crowded vegetarian/vegan market. Second, and more importantly, is that there are always people out there who take things to the extreme. When pseudoscience goes beyond dietary advice about eating raw vegetables, not eating meat, drinking wheatgrass dissolved in hydrogen-peroxide-spiked water, and almost worshipping the avocado; and is used, instead, to prey on and manipulate the vulnerable and most ill in society, that is when people get harmed, people die, and it becomes a true problem.

I have been criticised for lumping Bill Davies and Colin Campbell together with Robert Young. People asked me how I could compare two 'men of science' who were trying to make people healthier by changing their diets with a madman harbouring messianic delusions and who was trying to cure cancer. Remember, both Bill and Colin reference the alkaline way in their respective books. Yes, it is true that Robert took things to the extreme, where Bill and Colin did not. But it was all still on the same spectrum of pseudoscience. Both Bill and Colin claim that their respective 'grain-free' and 'plant-based' diets have miraculous curative effects similar to the claims made by Robert about the alkaline diet. Robert just shows what happens when it goes one not very large step further.

PART 4

A problem of our time

'One of the greatest problems of our time is that
many are schooled but few are educated.'

—Thomas More

'The significant problems of our time cannot be
solved by the same level of thinking that created
them.'

— Albert Einstein

'The question isn't, "What do we want to know about
people?" it's "What do people want to tell about
themselves?"'

— Mark Zuckerberg

CHAPTER 10

Eat like this and look like me

Like two billion other people in the world, I have a Facebook profile. I've got about 400 'friends', give or take. There is family of course (hi Mom!), and some are actual 'active friends', whom I meet, either regularly or periodically, depending on where in the world they live, and we go out for a meal, or a drink, or a movie; you know, friend stuff. Many others however, are 'Facebook friends', where because of the weird and slightly surreal world of social media, the last time you saw each other might have been twenty-five years ago at university. Yet I vicariously follow these 'Facebook friends' as they live their lives, and every so often I might 'like' the picture of their child's graduation from kindergarten to primary school, or when they move from Florida to Hawaii. Many of these friends will also follow along as I live my life, approving when I drink a fish-bowl-sized glass of pinot noir of an evening or 'hearting' the latest instalment of my son's food blog. Because all of this typically only happens within your circle of 'friends', it is all very low-key, allowing everyone involved to interact with each other, without the actual stress of having to have a relationship.

If Facebook acts as your virtual circle of friends, then think of Twitter as a virtual venue. It is used by many (too many, I feel), for instance, as a virtual pub or bar. What do people do at a pub? They occasionally get drunk, and sometimes end up shouting out random things to the room. These things could be deep and insightful, they may be funny or idiotic, but sadly they are too often misogynistic or racist or fascist, and then people will shout similar niceties back in return. The problem is, people will do exactly the same on Twitter, and forget that they are not yelling out in a room full of other drunk people, but are actually broadcasting to the world. Many have lost their jobs or even torpedoed entire careers because of an ill-judged tweet. I'm not a fan of this most popular aspect of Twitter. Yet I do have a Twitter account, and I'd like to think I don't shout unpleasantries to the drunken room. Rather, I use Twitter as a virtual convention or conference centre. I tweet almost exclusively in a professional capacity (I figure no one on Twitter cares what wine I drink) and 'in character', my character being an obesity geneticist and a BBC science presenter. I do say things to the room, and people will mostly respond positively, or at least constructively; but even at a conference, people sometimes spend a little too much time at the bar. A major problem with Twitter is that tone and nuance are difficult to achieve in 280 characters, and so discussions, such as they are, can become unnecessarily heated. On the positive side, the character limit does force you to crystallise your thoughts and be succinct, which can only be a good thing. Being succinct is a lost art . . . and yes I do realise I am living in a glasshouse and juggling a multitude of stones, while writing a 100,000 word book.

Then there is Instagram. Unlike its two older cousins above, where you might choose to post just text or a link, with or without an accompanying picture, in Instagram, you have to post a picture; in fact, it is all about the picture. Instagram was founded in 2010 by Kevin Systrom and Mike Krieger, when they started an iPhone photo-processing and sharing platform. It remained relatively niche, available only on Apple-based devices, until it was bought by Facebook in 2012. Other than making it available on all mobile platforms, Facebook left Instagram largely to its own devices. It has since become wildly successful, boasting 800 million monthly users with 500 million interacting with the app daily. Compare this to Twitter's 300 million or so users, of whom about 100 million tweet daily. It was the ubiquity of good-quality smartphone cameras that created the space for Instagram. Its revolutionary feature, since copied by many other apps, was the ability to 'process' your photos directly on your phone. With a few taps and swipes, you could crop your picture and add a sepia-toned filter, or blur out the background and convert it to monochrome, or you could even mimic the effect of a 'tilt-shift' lens or add a vignette or adjust contrast and saturation. It was, in effect, a stripped-down Photoshop for your phone. That was the brilliance. It is so very obvious now, because aside from professional photographers and graphic designers, did anyone actually know how to do anything else with Photoshop other than create a jpeg? Suddenly, anybody could take what used to be a run-of-the-mill snap, and instantly convert it into something cool, something beautiful, something worth sharing.

#INSTAGRAM

Ella Mills, aka 'Deliciously Ella', owes much of her success to the way she's woven her personal life and her brand together online. Her brand does have a presence on both Facebook and Twitter, but Ella's meteoric rise coincided with that of Instagram. These things are notoriously difficult to chart, but it is clear that Ella was one of the early drivers (if not THE driver) of sharing beautiful and polished pictures of her food on Instagram. She did this in conjunction with telling her personal story of healing by changing her diet. The power of her story, her anecdote, coupled with the power of the image was a heady mixture, and Ella now has more than 1.2 million followers on Instagram. If you examine her feed, you will see that the vast majority of the images on display are those of gorgeously photographed, artistic displays of plant-based food, and not a few of herself with her equally easy-on-the-eye husband, Matthew Mills. Where she has led, many now follow. Natasha Corrett of Honestly Healthy and the Hemsley Sisters, for example, both have more than 300 thousand followers.

Go to any food establishment in the world today, from a street-food vendor in Bangkok to a BBQ joint in Memphis Tennessee, to a Michelin-star restaurant in London's Soho and I guarantee you there will be diners photographing their food, adding a 'Gingham' filter, throwing a little vignette, adjusting the contrast and sharing it on Instagram. Some, perhaps even many of you, will find the practice annoying and even distasteful. At this moment, I will have to raise my hand and plead guilty to occasionally partaking in this slightly narcissistic food-photography foible.

Far from discouraging 'Instagramming', however, many establishments actually began to embrace it. For example, in 2017, London's Heathrow Airport, whose many food establishments feed over 75 million passengers that pass through its four terminals every year, actually appointed the food-writer Hemsley sisters as its 'Instagram Food Ambassadors'! This is a *bona-fide* job now, apparently. Jasmine and Melissa Hemsley, in a video that is available online, as well as on screens in a few of the nicer restaurants in Heathrow, give some helpful advice on how to make your plate look gorgeously Instagrammable. The screen I caught this on was in Gordon Ramsey's 'Plane Food' restaurant in Heathrow's Terminal 5. It was early in the morning, before 7 a.m., and I was enjoying my favourite breakfast, Eggs Benedict, before I had to hop on a flight to Israel.

Why, you might wonder, did Heathrow link up with the Hemsleys? Well, based on their own research, up to one in seven UK travellers has chosen a holiday destination based solely on food seen on Instagram. Before you scoff, consider this; if you type in three of the most popular food-related hashtags, #food, #foodie or

#foodporn into the Instagram search bar, you'll end up with more than half a billion hits. That is billion with a 'b'. Food is HUGE on social media, and because of its focus on pretty pictures, it is one of the biggest things on Instagram.

What is interesting is that the only other subject that competes with #food on Instagram is #fitness or #fitspo where you get pretty pictures of very pretty people, wearing not very much, sporting abs and quads and delts and gluts, and doing fit things. I say interesting because a large number of these scantily clad fit people also display the meals that they eat 'post-workout', that have presumably contributed to their sculpted bodies. Work out like me, eat like me, look like me.

I sigh when I look down at my own unsculpted body (I have a 'one-pack') and have to admit just a bit of envy . . . and I am certainly not alone.

CLEAN EATING THROUGH THE YEARS

Food crazes are not new to this decade, this century or even this millennium. Alan Levinovitz, author of *The Gluten Lie: And Other Myths About What You Eat* draws the interesting link between diet and virtually every religion. For instance, two of the major monotheistic religions, Judaism and Islam, have very strict food laws, with the Jewish diet governed by Kosher principles and Islam requiring food to be Halal. Even in Catholicism (and I speak as someone raised in a household that tipped their hats towards Rome), famously known for its rules and its ceremony but generally *laissez faire* when it comes to food, many practitioners today still won't eat any meat other than fish on Fridays. Besides guidelines for clean or right living, other religions have, in the past, claimed that eating a certain way would lead to the development of magical abilities (which sounds more familiar to some modern notions of food). Taoist monks rejected grains, undertaking what they called Bigu (辟谷) or Wugu (五谷), the prohibition of the five grains. According to Levinovitz, this lifestyle was promoted some 2,000 years ago, and those that undertook it were promised they would develop magical powers, such as resistance to disease, the power to fly and teleport and even to live for ever. The 'prohibition' later shifted from grains to meat, and then to the additional intake of supplements, but the promises stayed the same.[1]

The religious figures of the past have been replaced with those today that advocate equally restrictive diets, many of whom feature in this book: Bill Davis and his war on grains; Colin Campbell and Caldwell Esselstyn's plant-based evangelism; and Robert Young's alkaline living. Although no one is promising immortality or spontaneous flight (at least not yet), they all claim, and they all probably believe, as did the monks, that their specific restriction has the potential to cure not only diet-related illnesses, but ALL diseases. However, while these old white dudes (and they are all old white dudes) speak emotively and have published books on their dietary restrictions, it is the 'contemporary lifestyle gurus' that have amplified their messages, taking what essentially were niche restrictive diets, and repackaging and rebranding them as a lifestyle to the broader public. Social media, in particular Instagram and its power of image, has been the weapon of choice for these gurus to spread the message. At the time of writing, if you typed #cleaneating into Instagram, you'd get more than 36 million hits, #glutenfree 20 million hits, #plantbased more than 13 million and #detox more than 10 million. That is nearly 80 million pictures of Buddha bowls, quinoa and avocado salads, courgetti 'pasta', nut-milk cappuccinos (dude, please), kale smoothies and green juice.

SELLING SNAKE-OIL TO THE VULNERABLE

The people that are marketing these lifestyles are, by and large, pretty young ladies equipped with washboard abs, tiny pores, which incidentally never appear to clog, and large and dedicated social-media followings. One of the criticisms I received about the *Clean Eating* documentary was that I was being sexist by only focussing on attractive young women when talking about the lifestyle gurus. I understood the concern; however, I was simply reflecting the reality of the industry. For example, forty-two of the top fifty 'Fitstagrammers' are women.[2] More broadly, 60 per cent of influencers on Instagram are women, and the most popular category for paid content is lifestyle, including food and fitness.[3]

Yes, I did say industry, and it is one that is expanding at a rapid rate. Many celebrities-turned-entrepreneurs have also leapt on to the bandwagon, endorsing such magical creations as Amanda Chantal Bacon's Los Angeles-based 'Moon Juice', which is marketed as 'Adaptogenic beauty and wellbeing'. Nope, I have no idea what that means either.

Moon Juice is just the company name, it isn't a product itself but a group of products. If you look at their website, they claim:

'to celebrate the unadulterated, exquisite flavors and healing force of raw vegetables, fruits, petals, herbs, roots, nuts and seaweeds as daily nourishment, beauty tools and high-powered natural remedies.'[4]

For example, one of their products is 'Raw, activated Californian almonds', which comes in a 500g pack and retails for USD$25. That is an awful lot of money for almonds. I get the feeling that it's because, like many of their other products, they have been activated. This means that the almonds have been soaked in alkaline water which, and I quote, 'awakens the nuts' dormant properties, increasing digestibility and micronutrient, vitamin, and enzyme count'. Hmmm, I wonder what happens when these high-end alkaline-activated almonds reach our pH 1.5 stomach?

We are also encouraged to explore their organic pressed juices, Moon Milks (no idea what this is), Cosmic Provisions, the Moon Pantry and their Moon Dust collection (one can only imagine).

'Moon Juice represents a holistic lifestyle that goes far beyond juices, milks, and snacks.'[5] (Although when you strip it back, what they sell are very expensive juices, milks and snacks, as well as cosmetics.) 'It's a healing force, an etheric potion, a cosmic beacon for those seeking out beauty, wellness and longevity.'[6]

I'll just leave that there for you to cosmically contemplate briefly.

When you buy into these gurus, you are getting far more than just recipes or supplements or lotions. You are buying into a philosophy and a lifestyle. Gwyneth Paltrow's GOOP, for instance, is a website where millions of people visit to buy lifestyle items, such as coffee enemas (don't even), jade eggs for your 'yoni' (without getting too gynaecological, gentlemen, you don't have a 'yoni') and to obtain health 'advice'. GOOP recently felt the need to speak out on 'The mysteries of the thyroid'. The expert voice they rely on is a self-proclaimed 'Medical Medium' (yes, a medium) who, and I quote, 'can scan the body from afar, and with the help of "spirit" explain what ails or does not'.[7] Perhaps this, at long last, explained how *Star Trek*'s Dr 'Bones' McCoy's trusty medical Tricorder actually works!

The entire industry leverages the age-old trick of aspirational marketing, of course, linking lifestyle to health, to beauty and to being thin. For most celebrities and models, and those that have made their way to online-influencer status, their figure, complexion and looks are largely down to their genes, with a dash of surgery here and there. Their success has less to do with their diet and much more to do with their drive and work-ethic, perhaps, but most of all a healthy dose of privilege and luck. These influencers are redefining what self-care looks like and what it costs. Mostly, it's a lot of navel-gazing and pandering to the body's every fleeting mood and sensation, as if to miss the tiniest shift is somehow not being true to oneself (it is certainly completely self-obsessed). There are many people out there, without the benefits of privilege or 'skinny' and 'beautiful' genes, who are trying their best to become healthier, who are desperate to lose weight, but are having a really difficult time, and are consequently vulnerable to exploitation. None of the gorgeous gurus are vulgar enough to explicitly enunciate it, of course, but everything in their books and their websites and their Instagram posts screams out *'Eat like this and be healthy like me. Eat like this and be successful like me. Eat like this and look like me'*.

The reason I am bringing this up is that in this fat-shaming culture we live in, the majority of these 'influencers' are setting unhealthy goals, unreachable for most. They are selling snake oil to the vulnerable.

#SAUSAGEGATE

But surely following these celebrities and gurus on Instagram and vicariously looking into their wonderful lives is just like buying *Heat* or *OK!* magazine and other such tabloid offerings? You buy them, perhaps to look at the salacious paparazzi-obtained photos, ogle at the celebrity weight gain, sigh in envy at the weight loss, and read about divorces, surgeries and diets. It is all a bit of light entertainment, isn't it? Where's the harm, you party-pooper?

When I began making the *Clean Eating* documentary, I got myself an Instagram account. I figured if I was investigating the world, then I was going to have to try my best to insert myself into the world. But starting from literally zero was actually quite tough. The researcher on the programme was a razor-sharp young lass named Zoe Hunter Gordon, who was far more *au fait* with Insta than I was, and she devised a strategy for me. So first

I followed as many of the gurus that I could find; in addition, I searched for #cleaneating, #glutenfree, #plantbased, #detox and followed as many of the 'influencers' using these hashtags (which I defined arbitrarily as anyone with more than a thousand followers) as I could. I then spent a bit of time every day 'liking' everything posted by the gurus and influencers, in the hope that a few of them would follow me back. Finally, whenever I posted anything, for instance if I took a picture of a Deliciously Ella or Hemsley dish I had just tried, I would liberally hashtag the post with #eatarainbow, #poweredbyplants, #dairyfree, #traditionalfood *ad nauseum*. Because you search for posts on Instagram using these hashtags, then anyone interested in #eatarainbow posts, for example, would be able to find my picture. In my first eight days, I picked up about 300 followers, which was quite a way from Ella's 1.2 million, but hey, I was not an ex-model millionaire plant-based entrepreneur, so I figured it was a start.

One Sunday, as was usual, I made a cooked breakfast for my family. It was a pork sausage and a fried egg on a toasted English muffin, the kind used in Eggs Benedict. When placed next to a cup of tea, to my decidedly non-expert eye, it certainly looked quite photogenic. So I took a picture, made it look pretty with some processing, and put it up on Insta with the caption 'Sausage Yeo Muffin' (the name is trademarked, by the way), without giving it a second thought. It turned out to be a big mistake. Many of the people following me, of course, were in the Clean Eating world; that was the point of me starting the account after all. In the next couple of hours, I lost more than 10 per cent of my followers, because I posted the picture of a sausage. Someone actually commented acerbically, *'Thought you might be vegan, with all the food research you've done!'*, before summarily unfollowing me.

I had been judged and sentenced, harshly it would seem, for my love of sausages; or was it for my sausage photography? Both, I would have imagined.

DIGITALLY DRUNK

In life, rightly or wrongly, we are very often judged for what we look like, the accent we have, what we wear, what music we listen to and, yes, even the food we eat. It can be very unpleasant indeed when it happens in person. For the most part, however, while all kinds of thoughts, pleasant or otherwise, do percolate through our heads all of the time, societal norms still prevent most of us from being rude straight to someone else's face. It does happen in some (many?) people when their behaviour is disinhibited by alcohol. It can also happen sometimes when we lose our temper, and then there are others on the sociopathic spectrum for whom societal norms mean little; but in sobriety, it is thankfully relatively rare. Allowed to hide behind the anonymity of being online, however, and suddenly all bets are off. Social media appears to act like digital alcohol, freeing us to say things to strangers that we would never in a million years dare say to them in person.

While I had been an active social-media user before, this was the first time that I had put myself in a position to be judged by the public. This all turned out to be a valuable teaching moment and was also very eye-opening. But in this instance, the people judging me were not my 'peers,' with regards to our food philosophies. In fact, you might argue that our approaches to food could not have been further apart. So while what really did shock me was the immediacy of the response, I wasn't all that surprised with the actual result. How would I have felt, however, if those were my peers, sharing my food world view, from whom I was trying to seek approval?

Food and diet have always played a central role in religious and cultural identity. Also, all of us are, by definition, 'experts' at eating, given that we are alive. As a consequence, food choice, feeding behaviour and body size, all of which are outwardly visible, have always been subjected to judgement. Gluttony, after all, is one of the seven deadly sins, and many religions view fasting as a method of disciplining the body, delaying gratification for the afterlife. What social media has enabled is the democratisation of judgement. Everyone, should they choose, can now judge everyone else, without the constraint of having to consider the algorithms of societal niceties expected in face-to-face interactions. I only eat clean and real food; therefore I am MORE clean and real. If you don't, you must be dirty and fake. The moralisation of food is now amplified and fuelled by social media in secular culture just as intensely as it is alive in religion. Living healthily, such as it is, has become a moral achievement. Holding on to a few extra kilos and being overweight or (heaven forbid) obese has become the physical manifestation of greed, lack of self-control and laziness.

Keep in mind as well that Instagram is used by a far younger demographic than either Twitter of Facebook (which I presume is one of the reasons why Facebook bought Instagram to begin with). In 2017, for example, research showed that 76 per cent of thirteen- to seventeen-year-old American teens used Instagram.[8] Disturbingly, this recent rapid rise in the number of teens using social media has mirrored an increase in diagnoses of eating disorders in this same group. The UK National Health Service (NHS) reported that hospital admissions of people suffering from eating disorders doubled between 2012 and 2018, driven in part by social media, and with women under the age of twenty accounting for much of this increase.[9]

ORTHOREXIA

In 2017, Renee McGregor, a dietitian specialising in eating disorders, wrote a book entitled *Orthorexia*, in which she describes what happens when trying to eat healthily goes wrong, when healthy eating becomes an actual obsession. Dr Steven Bratman from San Francisco, who coined the term in 1996, described it thus on his website:

'Orthorexia is an emotionally disturbed, self-punishing relationship with food that involves a progressively shrinking universe of foods deemed acceptable. A gradual constriction of many other dimensions of life occurs so that thinking about healthy food becomes the central theme of almost every moment of the day, the sword and shield against every kind of anxiety, and the primary source of self-esteem, value and meaning. This may result in social isolation, psychological disturbance and even, possibly, physical harm.'[10]

Renee details four triggers for orthorexia.[11]

1) 'Feelings of being out of control.' When events in one's life are not going as they should be, a vulnerable person could turn to food as something they can find order in, something they can control.

2) 'Low self-esteem.' In this situation, a set of food rules to be followed, often obsessively, can sometimes provide a sense of success and fulfilment.

3) 'A need to be perfect.' Investigators have shown that orthorexia is strongly linked to perfectionism and body image attitudes. (In addition, a history of other eating disorders strongly predicts orthorexia nervosa.[12])

4) 'Lack of self-compassion.' Closely linked to the point above, when something is not perfect, there is an accompanied guilt, remorse and self-loathing.

Orthorexia is not officially recognised as an eating disorder in its own right, however. This is not because people doubt its existence; rather some argue that it is actually a variant of *anorexia nervosa* – *anorexia* from the Greek 'without appetite' and *nervosa* meaning 'obsession', so literally obsession with not eating. *Orthorexia* means 'correct appetite', so *orthorexia nervosa* is the obsession of correct eating.

Dr Angela Guarda, director of the Johns Hopkins Eating Disorders Program, was interviewed for an article on orthorexia that was published in the *Guardian* newspaper in 2015.[13] Angela said that eating disorders reflected the culture of the day. In the late 1990s, many of the anorexic patients that she saw were vegetarians. Whereas they now talk about eating exclusively organic food or say that they are lactose-intolerant and allergic to gluten, when their blood tests show that they are not.

Wherever you stand on the debate on whether orthorexia should or should not be considered a discrete eating disorder, suffice to say its symptoms are serious, chronic and go beyond a lifestyle choice. This obsession with healthy food can progress to the point where it crowds out other activities and interests, impairs relationships, and even becomes physically dangerous. Social media purports to celebrate food by making it look pretty and attractive. But to many, it drives fear for their choice of food, fear for their ability to prepare food, it drives fear of food. In those who are susceptible, it could trigger the onset of orthorexia, and even drive its progression.

In a study published in 2017, Pixie Turner and Carmen Lefevre from the Department of Clinical, Education and Health Psychology, University College London conducted an online survey of 680 social-media users who followed health-food accounts.[14] First of all, ALL 680 participants of the study were female (!), most of whom were under thirty. Try as they did, the investigators were simply unable to attract any males. The results were striking. First, they showed that higher Instagram usage was linked to increased symptoms of orthorexia, with no other social-media channels having this effect. Second, they showed that 49 per cent of this sample of female Instagram users who follow health-food accounts met the criteria for orthorexia! 49 per cent! This compares to the prevalence within the general population (which would include both males and females) of <1 per cent.[15] Remember that these social media 'celebrities', together, have many millions of followers. So while this was a relatively small study, these findings clearly highlight the impact that social media, in particular Instagram, can have on the psychological well-being of a significant proportion of young women.

THE NATASHA LIPMAN STORY

Consider, for example, the very public case of Natasha Lipman. Natasha was born with Elhers-Danlos syndrome, a connective-tissue disorder, which meant that her joints were prone to regularly and painfully dislocating. In addition, as if life had not dealt her a tough enough hand, she went on to develop two additional chronic conditions, an autonomic system issue called POTS (the same condition that Ella Woodward suffered from) and a histamine intolerance that left her with severe allergies to a number of foods including tomatoes. She felt so awful, with doctors and drugs having no apparent effect, that in early 2014, she turned to Doctor Google (where have we heard this story before?). As she scrolled through page after page, she found many young women suffering from similarly chronic conditions, but who had apparently cured themselves by turning to a plant-based diet. There they were, glowing, and posing next to the fruits and vegetables that had cured them. She fell for it hook, line and sinker. Natasha turned to a plant-based diet, and began taking pretty pictures of her food and documenting her experience on Instagram. For a time, Natasha felt better and she finally felt like she had some control over her health. As she had been inspired by other young women like her, other young women were inspired by Natasha, and her following began to grow. She ended up attracting international media attention. Even the BBC News wrote up a piece about how by changing her diet Natasha had begun to heal herself.[16] But while she initially found all of the social media, the followers, the media interest, very enticing, she also gradually found herself becoming obsessed with food. In a long, reflective and touching blog post in 2018, Natasha looked back on her story. She wrote:

'I was subsisting off of fruits and vegetables and almond butter. With the odd binge here and there. I became scared off non-organic produce. I became scared of organic produce that wasn't from Whole Foods. I spent nearly every minute thinking about food, preparing food, talking about food, researching food. I kept reading about these girls that were doing so well, and believed that I too could one day be one of the glossy girls laughing into a bowl of salad.'[17]

As the obsession grew and began to engulf Natasha, her health went into decline. But she convinced herself that the reason she was getting worse was that her diet was still not 'clean' enough. After all, that's one of the messages that's so pervasive in wellness: health is a choice. Make the right decisions and you'll be rewarded with health. What happens if you make the wrong decisions, though? What happens if you are not clean or real enough? What happens if you become dirty and fake? It is now clear that wellness can perpetuate self-blame amongst people, like Natasha, who was ill. Her diet became even more restrictive and extreme, which in turn worsened her health in a vicious cycle. Then one day, Natasha came to a damascene realisation that it was her restrictive, plant-based, clean diet that was killing her. It might have suited other people, but not her, certainly not someone in her condition. The problem was she now had quite a following on Instagram and her blog, so she had to pluck up the courage to let people know that she was going to eat meat again. This set off a whole torrent of abuse. She had betrayed the movement. Natasha wrote in her blog post:

'I cried the first time I ate pizza again because I felt like I could be poisoning myself. But I was also so happy. I slowly started to realise that the very small percentage of health benefit I was getting from such a strict diet wasn't worth the severely disordered eating I had developed. It took years to change, years to start reintroducing foods that I'd become pretty much brainwashed to believe were poisoning me.'

When I interviewed Ella for the *Clean Eating* documentary, I asked what her thoughts were on the dangers of social media driving disordered eating.

'You know what . . . I think there can be and I think it's up to us [social-media influencers] to be as responsible as we can be to do everything to allow people not to take it out of context. But to me that doesn't stop at food, that's the whole of social media and I think for the whole of social media, there's a collective body, there's a responsibility.'

THE BELLE GIBSON STORY

Then there was the far more controversial story of Belle Gibson. Belle was an Australian blogger and creator of the app and cookbook *The Whole Pantry*, which became a worldwide bestseller after she claimed that her 'clean' diet and alternative therapies reversed her terminal brain cancer. It was, of course, all too good to be true, but not before she had fooled millions and built up an enormous following. She later admitted she had never suffered from brain cancer and had in fact made the entire story up. Belle is now facing charges from the Australian government for false claims and contravening the country's consumer laws. Besides not actually having cancer, she also promised a portion of her profits would be donated to various causes and raised money with the help of her following on social media for charities that, in the end, never saw a penny.

This whole sordid tale inspired a book, *The Woman Who Fooled the World* by Beau Donelly and Nick Toscano, which charts Belle's rise and subsequent fall from grace. The deeper question asked by Beau and Nick, however, was how in the world did she fool so many people for so long? The publisher of Belle's recipe book, for instance, admitted to never fact-checking the story of her reversing brain cancer through diet and lifestyle, while eschewing conventional medical treatment.[18] Yet it was the headline story used to market the book. When Belle went on to encourage other cancer sufferers to do the same, no one questioned her, let alone criticised her. Instead, she was welcomed with open arms by not only the wellness community, but the media as well. The Angry Chef, who if you recall I shared a stage with at Food Matters Live, wrote in an opinion piece for The Pool:

'I suppose they were seduced by the dream, or afraid to burst the bubble. It is perhaps hard to critically interrogate a young woman when you believe she is suffering from a life-threatening disease. With the benefit of hindsight, even the most cursory glance at Gibson's story would have revealed holes, raised suspicions and invited questioning. And if just one person in the chain had done that, her poorly constructed lies would have collapsed like a house of cards.'[19]

We all love a good story. Who doesn't? But, desperate people, ill people, sad people, depressed people, will cling on to anything to try and help themselves feel even the tiniest bit better and in control.

LISTEN TO THE EXPERTS . . .

Whose responsibility is it to make sure people are doing what's right for them and making educated decisions about their food intake? Is it the people who are producing the content: the Ellas and, at the extreme end, the Belle Gibsons of the world? Or is it down to the people viewing the content? Which brings us to the 64-million-dollar-question. Why do so many people believe what clearly are 'alternative facts'? Ignorance and stupidity are answers that slip easily off the lips. If they only understood the science or the technology or did a bit more reading. However, it is easy to forget that we are all experts at something: driving, plumbing, cooking, window cleaning, in our own little patch of intellectual or technical real estate. Yet we all have 'faith' and believe in a multitude of things that we understand little about every single day. Take cars, for instance. Leaving aside all of you car mechanics and enthusiasts out there, how many of us truly understand how the brakes in our car work, let alone how the engine functions? How about planes? What keeps planes up in the air? Whenever I drive down the motorway past Heathrow, and see one of these giant aluminium beasts landing, all I can come up with is 'magic', which I am sure is unlikely to be the actual aeronautical explanation. Are you qualified to assess the primary climate-change data? Yet we all drive, or fly, and (most of us anyway) believe that humans have and continue to play a major role in global warming. We trust that other experts are doing their job and getting things right, and as a result, things happen, we get places, society functions.

The problem is, how does one tell an actual expert from a fake in this 'post-truth' era? While the consensus within the scientific community is that climate change represents a clear and present danger to our planet, there are (a very few) scientists that dispute this. Which scientist do you believe? The medical consensus is that not only are vaccines safe, but they play a critical role in preventing the spread of disease and hence ensuring the health of our children; yet it was a 'doctor' that published a paper (since discredited and retracted) claiming that vaccines cause autism. Most of us are not clinically trained, so which doctor should you believe? Then there are cardiologists and neurologists who are convinced that grains are poisoning us, and biochemists and surgeons that believe there is no safe dose of animal-based protein. Yet the scientific consensus simply does not support these claims. Whom should you believe?

THE MESSY TRUTH

The real unvarnished truth is that there are no easy answers. A big part of the problem is that scientists are not doing an effective enough job of communicating to non-experts; and I'm not just talking about the dissemination of facts and information. Scientists (me included) are not doing a good job of communicating how science works. What most people see are a bunch of white-coated individuals in their ivory towers arguing and disagreeing with each other. We've got to let people know that we are paid to argue and disagree with each other. Scientists are also criticised for changing their minds all of the time; nutritional guidelines used to say 'X', now it says 'Y'. Why don't you clowns make your mind up? We've got to inform the public that the very nature of evidence-based science is that ideas morph and change as new evidence emerges. Otherwise, progress comes to a grinding halt. Healthcare guidelines could be revised, and nutritional recommendations can often be reversed, which is, understandably, very frustrating to many. Yet it is what must be done in order to deliver the best possible treatment, in order to provide the best possible advice.

EAT LIKE THIS AND LOOK LIKE ME

Obesity and other diet-related illnesses are perceived to be simple problems of eating less and moving more; they are considered to be diseases of choice. In reality, the complex interactions between our genes and the environment mean that we all behave differently towards food, and hence there are no easy 'one-size-fits-all' solutions. That is the real and messy truth. There are no black or white answers, and even the greys constantly change their hue. Human beings simply do not like uncertainty, which is why many people, including those who are intelligent and well educated, find the conviction and confidence of the health gurus so attractive, so palatable, so easy to digest. Alternative-health gurus harness the language of medicine in order to sound authoritative. The real danger is that what they say is nearly always half-right. It is how pseudoscience works. Scientists, doctors, health professionals, dietitians and nutritionists, we all need to push back. All of us have a duty to engage in public conversations about health and diet; whether it is through speaking, or through the media, and yes, even (especially?) if it's through social media. If we do not, the discussion will be dominated by the beautifully and passionately uninformed, urging us to eat like them and look like them; who build trust only to sell false cures to the vulnerable who want to lose weight, who are trying their best to get healthier, who only want what is best for themselves and their families. The only way to combat this degradation of the value of truth is to be passionate about the truth. We have to find out the truth, tell the truth and call out untruths whenever and wherever we can.

CHAPTER 11

What's the right diet for you?

It was a cold Thursday in January, and I had just finished a day of filming in Camden, London. It was around 5.45 p.m. and the rush hour was in full swing. I made my way to the Camden Town Underground station to catch a Northern Line train south towards King's Cross station. When I got there, there was a large mass of people crowded around the entrance. I managed to squeeze my way to the front to see what was going on, only to find the accordion metal gate pulled shut. The station, with no explanation, was closed. Poo. I looked at my watch, knowing that the next express train back to Cambridge (and my dinner) was at 6.15 p.m., and King's Cross was only one tube stop away, maybe a three-quarters-of-a-mile walk. I had just about convinced myself that if I moved quickly, I could easily catch the train, when the heavens suddenly opened, and the rain came pouring down. Double poo. I had bags with me, my coat was not waterproof, I didn't have an umbrella and the temperature was hovering just around 4°C. At that moment, a black cab suddenly came round the corner, so I hailed it. The driver wound down his window.

'Where to, mate?'

'Can you take me to King's Cross?'

It was a very short journey through North London in rush-hour traffic, and I could see him running the algorithm in his head trying to figure out if this was actually worth the trouble.

'I don't know why, but they shut the bloody tube station. I was going to walk but then it started pissing down with rain. I'm trying to catch my train back to Cambridge, can you help?'

I tried my best puppy-dog eyes . . . fat lot of good that was going to do to convince a London cabbie.

'OK, OK, get in.'

It worked! Relieved, I jumped in.

A couple of minutes into the journey, with the windows steaming up from my wet clothing, he peered at me in the rear-view mirror and asked what I did up in Cambridge. I told him I studied food intake and obesity.

'Yeah? You know, I just started a f***ing diet two weeks ago. I've got two f***ing stone to lose.'

Well, hello, it seemed as if the cabbie–passenger relationship had suddenly entered a different phase.

'What kind of diet are you trying?'

'F***ing Slimming World.'

'Uh . . . is that like Weight Watchers?' I asked.

'Slimming World, f***ing Weight Watchers, they're all the f***ing same, innit? While you are weighing in weekly, you stay motivated to lose the f***ing weight. You don't wanna feel like a f***ing loser. The moment you stop, all the f***ing weight comes back on.'

He paused for breath to negotiate some traffic, and then peered at me in the mirror again.

'That's the problem with all these f***ing diets . . . they only work when you are f***ing on them.'

I nearly killed myself f***ing laughing. But he was, of course, entirely correct.

The rest of the journey went on in a similar vein, throughout which I was thoroughly entertained. The cab fare came to £6.50 and I tipped him a pound. I even made the 6.15 p.m. train.

This encounter got me thinking about some of the other diets available that actually do 'work' in terms of either weight loss or improvement of health. Are there any that are actually 'better' than others? Is there a 'right' diet to be on?

'RIGHT DIET'

While I had previously been interviewed as a 'talking head', it wasn't until 2015 that I had my first significant foray into communicating science on television. Together with three of my colleagues from the Universities of Cambridge and Oxford, I participated as an 'expert' in a three-part BBC series called *What's the Right Diet for You?*, following the trials and tribulations of seventy-five obese volunteers looking to lose weight. As my favourite taxi driver of all time said (I am paraphrasing from his colourful vernacular), any diet that gets you to eat less will lead to weight loss; however, if you stop the diet, the weight will, rather depressingly, invariably find its way back on. Why? Because weight loss, even a few pounds, is sensed as a big red danger signal, causing your body to push back by increasing metabolic efficiency and appetitive drive. So if you stop whatever diet you were on, and go back to how you were eating, your weight will soon climb back to where it was before you began the diet.

In view of this depressing fact, the programme asked whether knowing something about the differences in the biology under-lying our feeding behaviour could lead to the development of personalised dietary strategies, possibly resulting in a greater chance of us sticking to a diet and hence keeping the weight off. There are, of course, innumerable factors influencing people's eating behaviour. But we needed to start somewhere, so we began by screening more than 200 individuals for a myriad of different genetic, anthropometric, psychological and biochemical charac-teristics, eventually ending up with three groups of twenty-five, each with different and distinct reasons why they eat more than others.

The first group we called 'Feasters'. (The names of the three groups, incidentally, were foisted upon us by the producers, so that the audience could more easily follow what was going on and possibly even allow them to identify with a given behaviour.) Professor Fiona Gribble, a close colleague of mine from Cambridge (we are office neighbours), and an international expert on gut biology, found that this group produced lower levels of gut hormones after a meal, in particular, one called GLP1. Higher levels of gut hormones are normally a signal of fullness, so lower levels meant it was possibly more difficult for these individuals to stop eating. The second group we called 'Emotional Eaters'. As the name suggested, members of this group, who were identified by Paul Aveyard, a professor of behavioural medicine from Oxford, tended to eat in response to negative emotions such as anxiety, depression or stress. As a geneticist, however, I had a particular interest in the third group, which we called the 'Constant Cravers'. As I have discussed at the beginning of this book, it is unequivocal that genes play a role, to differing degrees, in influencing ALL of our bodyweights; the Constant Cravers, however, carried more genetic risk factors, making them feel slightly hungrier all the time (hence the name), leading them to eat more than others.

Armed with all of this information, Professor Susan Jebb, a nutritional scientist *par excellence* from Oxford, then made an initial attempt to design diets aimed at tackling the specific feeding behaviour characteristics of each group. This was a true 'experiment'; not in the sense that it was properly controlled (which it wasn't), but that no one had ever tried it before on this scale, and in front of the television cameras to boot.

A GLYCAEMIC INDEX FEAST

Because the 'Feasters' had a lower level of gut-hormone secretion in response to food, in theory that should either make them feel less full or take longer to get full. It was the latter possibility that gave them the moniker of a 'Feaster'. So whatever the dietary strategy, it needed to focus on boosting gut-hormone release. We ended up placing the 'Feasters' on a high-protein and low glycaemic index (GI) carbohydrate diet. As I have already discussed, because proteins take longer to digest than fat and carbs, hence are less calorically available, they end up travelling further down the gut, which, due to hormonal release, makes you feel fuller.[1] The purpose of increasing the amount of protein eaten was therefore to try and increase gut-hormone release. How about the 'glycaemic-index' element?

The glycaemic index or GI is a rating system used to show how quickly carbohydrate-containing foods affect blood glucose levels. The highest GI food is, by definition, sugar, which is almost completely calorically available and therefore very quickly makes it into the bloodstream. Caloric availability, if you recall, is the amount of calories that can actually be extracted during the digestion process, as opposed to the total number of calories that are locked up in the food. The GI rating of sugar is therefore set at the maximum rating of 100, with all other foods indexed against that number. The principle of the GI diet is to try and keep the rise in blood glucose after a meal as slow and steady as possible, by eating foods that take longer to digest and hence release their carbohydrates more slowly; so-called low-GI foods. The longer a particular food takes to digest . . . yup, you've got it, the further down the gut it will go before being absorbed, and the fuller you will feel. Low-GI foods are anything with a score of 55 or less, medium-GI foods 56–69, and high-GI foods will have a score above 70. Broadly speaking, the higher the GI of a food, the more rapidly it is digested, so you can't really discuss GI without considering caloric availability.

Any foods which contain a lot of refined carbohydrates, either as free sugars or as refined white flour, or have very little fibre, are going to fall into the high-GI category. These are of course anything sugary, and also white bread, white rice and potatoes. Medium- and low-GI foods include some fruit (depending on how sugary they are) and vegetables, pulses and whole grains, with the fibre and protein (in the pulses) slowing down their digestion.

It does all sound very straightforward, until you look a bit closer at the many GI food lists that are available online, and realise, perhaps unsurprisingly, that foods with a high GI are not necessarily unhealthy and not all foods with a low GI are healthy. So, many sweet fruits that are lower in fibre, such as watermelon and sweet root vegetables such as parsnips are high-GI foods; whereas a carrot cake has a lower GI value than either. Why would this be the case, given that the cake is packed full of sugar and would almost certainly have been made with refined white flour?

The weakness of the GI value system, is that levels are calculated based on a particular food being eaten in isolation. Case in point, cooking foods in fat or protein reduces caloric availability, slowing down the absorption of carbohydrates and therefore lowering their GI. Potato crisps or chips, for example, because they are fried in fat, have a lower GI than boiled or baked potatoes. I love, LOVE, all variations of fried potatoes . . . but sadly, no one can say, certainly not with a straight face, that a crisp or chip is healthier than a boiled potato; thus, they do have to be eaten in moderation. Another example is chocolate, which has a medium GI even though it is full of sugar, because of its fat content. How about the carrot cake? Well, while it is full of white flour and sugar, it also has some fibre (carrots and sultanas . . . but I would hesitate to count it as one of our five-a-day), as well as a significant amount of fat (cream-cheese icing, butter and milk) and protein (nuts, cream cheese, milk and eggs) in it, thereby lowering its total GI.

Another added complexity is that the ripeness of food will also influence its GI. This is particularly true for bananas. Green bananas (an acquired taste) compared to yellow bananas (perfection) compared to brown bananas (chuck it in a cake with some walnuts already!), have hugely different sugar content and thus vary in their GI. Finally, the absolute amount of carbs you eat has a bigger effect on blood glucose levels than GI alone. Pasta, for example, has a lower GI than watermelon, but it also contains a lot more carbohydrates than watermelon. Thus, if you eat similar amounts, in weight, of either of these two foods, the pasta will end up having a bigger impact on your blood glucose levels.

The bottom line is, considering the GI of carbohydrate-containing foods is a great way to find healthier, higher-fibre and lower-sugar options. However, focussing only on the GI of foods, without taking into account other aspects, could result in an unbalanced diet, high in fat and calories, which could lead to weight gain, which is presumably not why you would embark upon this diet to begin with!

EMOTIONAL GROUP SUPPORT

The 'Emotional Eaters' tended to eat in response to negative emotions, including stress. The 'stress' I refer to here is not the acute 'a tiger is about to eat me' type of stress. That has a universal response of stopping whatever you happened to be doing at that point and running away as fast as possible. Rather, I am referring to chronic stress, such as you might face at work trying to meet a deadline or during exam time when you were at school. What is interesting is that not everyone eats more in response to this type of chronic stress. In fact, there are probably just as many people who eat less or stop eating when stressed. We know that it is the hormone cortisol that is released from the adrenal gland when you are stressed, but we don't really know why people respond to this same hormone in diametrically opposite ways.

One plausible explanation is that because stress is, well, stressful, and therefore unpleasant, our opposite responses represent different strategies to make us feel better. So I, for instance, eat when I'm stressed, but end up craving specific types of food that I find comforting. At the risk of backing myself into a stereotype, my ultimate comfort food, when I am stressed, is a big bowl of noodles. It can be chow mein or hofun or Japanese ramen or Vietnamese pho, but it's got to be noodles. These particular foods seem to tickle a part of my brain that makes me feel better. For others, however, food probably doesn't do the trick; it may have to be running or cycling, or it may require a huge adrenaline surge, such as from bungee jumping or base-diving, that then triggers parts of their brain to relieve stress (you know who you are!). What would happen if people who eat because of stress could find something else to do that made them feel better? Would they then end up eating less?

It was for this reason that the Emotional Eaters were placed on a combination of cognitive behavioural therapy and group support. The thought here was that the cognitive behavioural therapy would help the volunteers with strategies to find other things to overcome stress, without necessarily turning to food. As for group support, well, being with 'like-minded' individuals provides encouragement and activates the motivation areas of the brain. We have all been in the situation of planning a run or a workout at 8 a.m. on a Sunday morning. We're all gung-ho the night before, but as the alarm goes off at 7.30 a.m. on Sunday morning, our motivation has suddenly evaporated faster than a drop of water in a hot pan. If you've made plans to work out with a buddy, however, you are far more likely to force yourself out of bed, because you don't want to let him or her down. Equally, it is simply easier to stick with a weight-loss plan when you have support and can share tips and motivation, and have to weigh in every week.

In one study, researchers looked at the effectiveness of 'Weight Watchers'" group support versus a self-help approach involving two meetings with a dietician and some printed materials.[2] In the first year, the Weight Watchers participants, on average, lost roughly 4kg (10 pounds) compared to 1.3kg (3 pounds) in the self-help group. By the end of the second year, both groups had regained some weight. But while the self-help group returned pretty much to their starting weight, the average Weight Watchers participant managed to keep off 3kg (6 pounds). The problem of course, is what is the effectiveness long term? You can already see that in the second year of the study, weight is beginning to be regained, probably because their bodies have begun to push back by reducing energy expenditure and increasing hunger. As was so eloquently delineated by my favourite taxi driver (once again I am paraphrasing), you have to stay on the programme in order to keep the weight off. And as with all approaches, they are not going to work for everyone. Some will embrace with open arms the social element and find motivation in the competitive weigh-ins; they may not be sold or marketed as being competitive, but they are after all public weigh-ins. Many, however, find the whole process so abhorrent, making them feel ashamed because they haven't achieved their weight-loss target for the week, that it will stress them out, driving them to eat even more! So it is most certainly not suited to all.

INTERMITTENT FASTING FOR CRAVERS

Finally, there were my team of obese volunteers, the genetically predisposed 'Constant Cravers'. We had screened the original group of 200 people for the top 25 of the 100 genes associated with BMI that I spoke about at the end of Chapter 2.[3] The 25 genes we chose were the ones with the largest impact on average BMI. So, for example, the gene with the biggest effect on weight on the list was called Fat Mass and Obesity Related Transcript or FTO.[4] Like with all the genes we screened, all of us have FTO. Some of us, however, have inherited a slightly different version of FTO, which increases our risk for becoming obese. If you carry one copy of the risk variation of FTO, you are on average 1.5kg heavier, and if you carry two copies, then you are on average 3kg heavier. And so it went down the list of 25, with smaller and smaller effects on BMI. From there, we calculated a genetic 'risk score'. Consider each genetic variant having a possible score of 2 (two copies of the risk allele), 1 (one copy) or 0 (two copies of the protective allele). With 25 genes, that is a potential maximum risk score of 50 (25 x 2) and a minimum of 0, although most of us will have an average risk score, that being how genetics works. The 25 people with the highest risk scores were then selected for the study. The biology of the system tells us, simplistically, that people who are at a higher genetic risk of obesity are slightly 'hungrier' all of the time, thus their name, the 'Constant Cravers'.

Of all the three groups, this one was, in many ways, the weakest one. Why? Because although the genetic risk score was an empirical number, and all 25 did indeed have a high genetic risk, each individual's mix of genetic variations that led to the score was different. In other words, each of the 25 Constant Cravers had their own unique reasons that led them to eat more. It also means that it is very difficult to quantify how much hungrier the group is, because each individual will also have different levels of hunger. This is a key point that I will address in detail in the next chapter.

Because all of the Constant Cravers were different, picking a single 'personalised' diet for them all was also proving difficult. The strategy was therefore to think about how to best tackle the constant hunger. In the end, the Constant Cravers were placed on an 'intermittent-fasting' diet. There are a number of variations of intermittent fasting, with the three most common ones being:

a) *Whole-day fasting* — which is 1–2 days per week of up to 25 per cent of daily caloric requirements, with no food restriction on the other days;

b) *Alternate-day fasting* — where people alternate between days of no restriction with days consisting of one meal providing around 25 per cent of daily caloric requirements and

c) *Time-restricted feeding* — where, for instance, you may eat all of your meals in an 8-hour window (typically, this window can range from 6–10 hours) during the day, and fast the remaining 16 hours.

Susan Jebb had chosen the whole-day fasting option, where for two days out of every seven, the Constant Cravers had to limit their intake to 800 calories with few or no carbohydrates, and to eat normally for the remaining five days. We reasoned that because this group felt hungrier all the time, it would be easier to stick to a diet if they could focus on it just two days a week. This plan was a variant of the '5:2' diet as popularised by BBC health journalist Dr Michael Mosley in his book *The Fast Diet*. The original 5:2 recommends consumption of a 'normal' number of calories five days a week and then, for two, non-consecutive days, 500 calories for women and 600 for men. Susan tweaked it by placing the two 'fast' days consecutively, and having dieters consume 800 calories but with minimal to no carbohydrates. Her rationale was that on the first of the two consecutive low-carb fasting days, a dieter should be able to deplete much of the stored carbohydrates (glycogen), such that on the second fasting day, the body would begin burning fat, in effect going into ketosis. It was a 'ketogenic diet lite', clearly nowhere near as extreme as its big brother.

There is no doubt that intermittent fasting is suited to some people as a weight-loss strategy. I certainly don't consider it a 'fad diet', because you are not buying or eating anything out of the ordinary, and you are not restricting entire food groups for no reasons. You are just eating a little bit less of everything, but in a timetabled fashion. As long as you don't overcompensate on the non-fasting days, you will go into calorie deficit, which will lead to weight loss. The BIG question is whether there is any additional benefit to doing it by intermittent fasting, as opposed to reducing calories in a myriad of other ways? In terms of weight loss, no. The research is unequivocal that a calorie deficit is a calorie deficit, no matter how you achieve it. For instance, a randomised clinical trial among 609 overweight adults, showed no difference in the amount of weight lost over twelve months between those on a low-carbohydrate diet (−6.0kg), versus those on a low-fat diet (−5.3kg).[5] There were also no differences in other metabolic measurements such as insulin sensitivity. Thus, intermittent fasting, like going on a low-fat or low-carb diet, is simply a strategy that better suits some people to achieve a calorie deficit and hence lose weight. For some, focussing all one's efforts on a couple of days' severe calorie restriction is the way to go, especially if you want to carry on socialising with friends and family. For others, however, their temperament may be better suited to implementing a moderate restriction but every day. Of course, lifestyle can also get in the way; so shift-workers who are working seven days on and seven days off for instance, could find intermittent fasting difficult.

How about other benefits to metabolic health beyond that obtained from weight loss? This is less clear. There are some who argue that intermittent fasting mimics the food environment that humans would have experienced during much of their hunting and gathering existence prior to agriculture. It is part of the 'paleo' argument, that since this is what we were adapted to, a feast and famine environment of periodic food availability, it must be better for us than constant food availability. It is true that many studies in mice do show an association between periodic fasting and small improvements in both metabolic and brain health, when compared to simple overall calorie restriction. Intermittent fasting is argued to result in periodic ketosis, and that the body benefits from a switch of fuel from glucose to ketones every so often. It is an attractive proposition that makes some evolutionary sense, and I am certainly not dismissing it out of hand. However, high-quality randomised control trials in humans comparing intermittent fasting to overall calorie restriction are, to date, limited. One study has shown that intermittent vs continuous calorie restriction shows some positive effects on glucose levels after a meal, as well as lipid metabolism following matched weight loss in overweight and obese participants.[6] But it was a small study, so I think this is still a work in progress. Our own attempt at deploying this approach, for instance, was to achieve a caloric deficit, rather than in the belief that it would lead to any additional metabolic benefits.

But intermittent fasting, as I've described, is certainly not bad for you, although it won't suit everyone's lifestyle or temperament. You should seek medical advice if you choose to embark upon such a diet if you are pregnant, because in some, fasting can be seen as a stressor, which you want to avoid when pregnant. Instead, pregnant women are advised to eat healthily and regularly. Intermittent fasting if one has type 1 diabetes can also be tricky because of the delicate balance that needs to be achieved between the amount of insulin that needs to be injected and the amount of food that has been eaten. It is also best avoided if one has a history of eating disorders that involve unhealthy self-restriction, such as anorexia, orthorexia or bulimia nervosa.

IMPERFECT PERSPECTIVE

The initial results from the first three months, which were filmed for the programme, were encouraging, with all three groups losing copious amounts of weight. Only time will tell, of course, if the weight will stay off in the long run. Did this new, more 'personalised' approach make it easier to stick to a diet? Well, in truth, we don't know. With it being a 'demonstration study' (as opposed to a proper trial) set up for television, it wasn't conducted over a long enough period of time, it didn't have proper controls and had too few participants to show anything conclusive. Did we, for that matter, even select the appropriate diets for the different groups? But it was a start. As I said, there are many, many more than three different 'groups' out there, and the more specific we can get in determining the biology of a person, the better our chances of success at designing a diet they are more likely to stick to. The proper randomised controlled studies, which the 'Right Diet' programme certainly was not and never pretended to be, need to be done.

But to be clear, imperfect though it was, I never regretted for one moment, and continue to be proud of, my involvement in making the programme. It was, after all, a series broadcast in prime time, portraying obese people sympathetically and without judgement, while at the same time communicating that there was a biological basis to the control of food intake and bodyweight. I am a molecular geneticist and so my 'day job' is largely lab-based, moving small volumes of colourless liquids from one tube to another, and then analysing data on computers. Thus, from my own personal perspective, by far the most precious thing I gained from my 'Right Diet' experience was my interaction with the obese participants. Of the 75 original volunteers that took part in the 'Right Diet' programme, 67 are part of a private Facebook group, which I was invited to join. Here, they continue their struggle (and it is a struggle) to lose weight and try to keep it off together; sharing successes, failures, marriages, babies and divorces. It has been an honour to sit quietly in the corner of this group, almost as a voyeur. This has provided a face to the problem and given me much-needed perspective; that beyond the often myopic view of lab-based academic science and publications and grants, there are human beings who are suffering; who are not only debilitated by obesity, but are also accused of lacking will-power, being lazy and being bad. In turn, this perspective provided impetus and motivation to my own research. It also crystallised my message and thereby made me far more effective in communicating it to the public. In fact, it was this personal experience, coupled with the exposure that I received because of my participation with the 'Right Diet' programme, that provided me with the opportunity to begin presenting science documentaries for the BBC.

IMPROVED HEALTH WITHOUT WEIGHT LOSS? – THE MEDITERRANEAN DIET

As we have discussed at length in this book, there are many diseases linked to obesity, and we know that losing a large amount of weight reverses type 2 diabetes in most (but not all) people and reduces the risk for all the other diseases. Are there diets out there, however, which do get you to become healthier without necessarily getting you to lose weight?

It was the end of November in 2016, and I was in Cordoba, Spain, to speak at a conference called 'New Frontiers in Obesity Research'. As you might imagine, it was just the kind of thing that floated my boat. There were symposia on adipocyte (fat cell) biology, the brain and obesity, the microbiome and obesity and new drug targets in obesity. And even though (or maybe given that) it was an obesity meeting, the food was excellent. We had a wonderful 'Tapas Night', where the highlight for me was a fabulous dish made with Iberico pork, which comes from a traditional breed of Spanish pig that has been raised on acorns. It is like Wagyu beef in terms of its marbling, and simply melted in my mouth. In fact, my mouth is beginning to water again simply writing about it! Sorry, where was I again? Oh yes, the meeting.

Aside from the food however, the real scientific highlight for me was to hear Dr Jordi Salas-Salvadó from Reus, in Catalonia, Spain, speak. Jordi was one of the investigators in the Prevención con Dieta Mediterránea, or PREDIMED, consortium; a group of Spanish clinicians and scientists who set up a landmark study examining the role of the Mediterranean diet in the prevention of disease.

There are certain populations that famously do live longer than others. The Japanese and Scandinavians are classic examples, and efforts have been made to understand why this might be the case. Genetics will clearly play a large role, but the diets of these populations are also the subject of scrutiny. One other important group notable for their health and longer life-spans are those living along the shores of the Mediterranean, and in recent years, considerable efforts have been put into studying the benefits of their diet.

The traditional Mediterranean diet is characterised by a high intake of olive oil, fruit, nuts, vegetables, grains and cereals. It encourages a moderate intake of fish and poultry and a low intake of dairy products, red meat, processed meats, and sweets. Finally (and most importantly?), wine can be consumed in moderation, but with meals. There have been many previous observational studies showing that risk of cardiovascular disease goes down with adherence to a Mediterranean diet. The PREDIMED consortium however, conducted a randomised trial to test the effectiveness of two variations of the Mediterranean diets (one supplemented with extra-virgin olive oil and another with nuts), as compared with a control diet (dietary advice and a low-fat diet), on the prevention of cardiovascular disease.[7]

It was a large study with 7,447 Spanish participants, men and women between the ages of fifty-five and eighty, all of whom either had type 2 diabetes, smoked, had high blood pressure or had elevated LDL (so-called bad) cholesterol. In other words, the participants all had a high risk of, but did not yet have, cardiovascular disease at enrolment to the study. They were randomised to one of three diets: a Mediterranean diet supplemented with a litre of extra-virgin olive oil per week (no, that is not a typo and yes, it is a litre of olive oil, per person per week; this is next-level stuff, no messing about); a Mediterranean diet supplemented with 30g/day of mixed nuts (for those of you taking notes for your next trip to the supermarket, this was composed of 15g of walnuts, 7.5g of hazelnuts, and 7.5g of almonds; and adds up to 900g of mixed nuts per month); or a control diet (a standard American Heart Foundation low-fat diet). You might wonder why the control diet was 'low-fat' and not an unhealthy one, surely that would have produced a far larger benefit? True. But the answer is that ethically, you cannot recruit people at high risk of heart disease and feed them doughnuts! That's the kind of thing that could get you into all sorts of problems.

The participants were not asked to limit portion sizes or to exercise more. They were on the diets between three and seven years, which is a very long time! How many of you have managed to stick to a diet for a few months, let alone years? The primary measured endpoints for the study were the rate of major cardiovascular events, i.e. heart attacks, stroke, or death from cardiovascular causes; all pretty hard endpoints, I think you'll agree, not subject to interpretation.

So what were the scores on the door? Bottom line was that folks on either the extra olive oil or extra nut versions of the Mediterranean diet had a 30 per cent reduction in major cardiovascular events compared to those on the regular 'low-fat' diet. Thirty per cent! Keeping in mind that cardiovascular disease remains the most common cause of death in the world, accounting for 32 per cent of ALL deaths in 2013.[8] The really interesting thing in this case, was that the key driver in protecting against heart disease did not appear to be weight loss (although weight loss would have independent protective effects), because there were no significant weight differences between the groups. Rather, it did appear to be the Mediterranean diet *per se*.

Now for the crucial question; why and how did it work? The short answer is – we still don't know. The key difficulty in this study was that unlike in a drug trial, where the absence and presence of the drug in question is the only variable, PREDIMED was testing an entire diet versus another. So trying to work out which component of the Mediterranean diet was imparting a protective or preventative effect has proven difficult. Could it be the reduction of red and processed meats? Is it the lowering of the consumption of dairy products? Could it perhaps be the increase in fish intake? Or whole grains? Perhaps it was the wine (one can always hope)? It is very likely that the addition of extra-virgin olive oil and nuts had a major role to play. The main type of fat found in olive oil is monounsaturated fatty acids, while nuts have a high content of both monounsaturated and polyunsaturated fatty acids, and higher consumption of unsaturated fats has been clearly linked with lower mortality.[9] However, it is most likely to be the whole diet acting in concert, the reduction in red and processed meats (and by extension saturated fats) together with the addition of fish, whole grains, olive oil and nuts, that produces the maximal protective effect against disease.

PITFALLS IN PIOPPI

There are a few things to think about before you start knocking back shots of olive oil. First, the amount of olive oil suggested, one litre a week, seems incredible to a Mediterranean diet novice like me. Previously, I think I might have gone through a litre a month for the whole family! After hearing that talk by Jordi in Cordoba, I began consuming more of both olive oil and nuts. It is certainly far easier to consume 30 grams of nuts a day! There is the real issue of how to deliver such a diet here in Cambridge, UK, or for that matter in Dallas, Texas. In Cambridge, the only fish that is available consistently and relatively cheaply is salmon, which I love, but can I eat it twice a week every week? For the Spanish participants of the study, the Mediterranean diet was their standard diet, so they didn't need to be familiarised with it. Whereas in order to increase uptake of such a diet in the UK or in large swathes of the US, more work will need to be done to improve literacy on the foods in the diet, and to also work with supermarkets to carry more Mediterranean produce. Finally, there is a risk of excess calorie intake because specific amounts of foods and portion sizes are not emphasised, particularly if you are drinking copious amounts of olive oil and munching on nuts, which could lead to weight gain. However, it is important to note that, probably in part due to the higher intake of olive oil and less processed food, consuming a Mediterranean diet seems to be more satiating, and the PRED-IMED study certainly showed no significant weight gain by the participants. It's just important to keep it in mind, I feel.

There are, of course, regional variations in the Mediterranean diet, which can be seen as you compare and contrast the Spanish, French, Italian and Greek interpretations of Mediterranean cuisine, for instance. But whole grains, fish, olive oil and nuts tie them all together. The oddest interpretation of the diet, however, has come from cardiologist Aseem Malhotra and filmmaker Donal O'Neill, in a book they published in 2017 called *The Pioppi Diet*.[10] Pioppi is a small Italian village, and it is actually UNESCO-protected as the 'home of the Mediterranean diet'. Thus, it is perfectly natural that you might have thought, since they named their diet plan 'Pioppi', that Aseem and Donal may have stayed true, or at least within shouting distance of its Mediterranean roots. But no. There is a slightly generic 'lifestyle' component to this diet, which involves walking at least 30 mins a day, sleeping at least 7 hours and being less stressed, which, to be fair, is hardly controversial. It is in the dietary component of their plan that oddities emerge. Yes, olive oil and nuts do indeed play a role, but there the similarities end. They encourage you not to fear all types of fat. Saturated or unsaturated, eat all you want! They encourage the consumption of copious amounts of red meat. They seem to suggest you replace milk with coconut milk. They do suggest wine with food . . . but then they ban all carbs. Like, everything from free sugars all the way to complex carbs tied up in whole grains.[11] Go cold turkey, they say! All of it begins to make a bit more sense when you realise that Aseem and Donal are both ardent advocates of the low-carb, high-fat diet.[12] Now I have discussed low-carb, high-fat diets in detail in Chapter 4, and there is undoubtedly a market for them, and even some evidence that they may be effective in the management of some people with type 2 diabetes. My issue here is surely by using the name of the village, you are implying a specific geographical relevance to the diet? Some sense of UNESCO-protected space? No one in Pioppi, however, is on a low-carb diet, because they are all Italians, and would possibly kick you out of Pioppi should you try to take away their pasta and bread. No one in Pioppi is going to, as suggested by Aseem and Donal, replace a traditional pizza base with a slice of cauliflower (surely it wouldn't be a pizza then, but a kind of tomato-y cauliflower cheese?).[13] Finally, there are no coconut trees in Pioppi, just sayin'.

DASH

Another diet where the primary aim is not weight loss is the 'Dietary Approaches to Stop Hypertension' or DASH diet. Hypertension is the clinical term for high blood pressure. The DASH diet consists primarily of fruits and vegetables, low-fat milk, whole grains, fish, poultry, beans and nuts. It recommends reducing salt, foods and beverages with added sugars, red meat and saturated fat. Thus, it has many similarities with the Mediterranean diet, but without the explicit addition of olive oil. It is also far more prescriptive, with the diet suggesting a specific number of servings of the recommended foods listed above. For instance, if one were to be consuming 2,000 calories a day on the DASH diet, this would translate to about 6–8 servings of grains (whole grains recommended), 4–5 servings vegetables, 4–5 fruits, 2–3 low fat dairy foods, 2 or fewer 85-gram servings of meat, poultry, or fish, 2–3 servings of fats and oils, and 4–5 servings of nuts, seeds, or dry beans per week. It also advises limiting foods with added sugars to 5 servings or fewer per week. The serving sizes of each of these food groups are different, and are detailed on a number of different websites, including one from the National Heart, Lung and Blood Institute, which is a part of the US National Institute of Health,[14] and seems as reputable a source as any!

The problem with the diet is that it requires each person to plan their own daily menus based on the allowed servings, which are not intuitive, and I just feel that folks who are not used to meal preparation and cooking will need a lot of help with DASH. That being said, numerous studies show wide-ranging health benefits of the DASH diet. For one thing, it 'does what it says on the tin' and is effective at lowering blood pressure.[15] DASH has also been found to lower the risk of a painful inflammatory condition called gout, in susceptible individuals.[16] (As an aside, most people still associate

gout with rich greedy Dickensian men, like in *Oliver Twist*. However, we now know that there are powerful genetic drivers that
increase susceptibility to this very painful disease.) There is also
evidence of DASH reducing the risk of cardiovascular disease.[17]

NUDGE

Then there are evidence-based changes – actually, change is
too strong a term, more like tweaks, nudges, even, that can be
made to improve aspects of your own and your family's diet, that
don't even involve dieting at all. 'Nudge' is in fact a fully fledged
concept in behavioural science and economics, which proposes
positive reinforcement and indirect suggestions to try to influence
decision-making of groups and individuals. A classic example of
'nudge' was when the guy in charge of keeping the loos clean at
Amsterdam's Schiphol Airport (if you've ever been to Schiphol,
there are many loos indeed) etched an image of a housefly in the
men's urinals, in an effort to, shall we say, 'improve aim'. It ended up
working a treat and lowering cleaning bills, so much so that the fly
(or flying saucer, or skull and crossbones, or flower) in the urinal
is now much mimicked throughout the world. It was a theory first
mooted by Richard Thaler in the book *Nudge – Improving Decisions about Health, Wealth and Happiness*, which he published
with Cass Sunstein in 2008. In it they write:
'A nudge, as we will use the term, is any aspect of the choice
architecture that alters people's behavior in a predictable way
without forbidding any options or significantly changing their
economic incentives. To count as a mere nudge, the intervention
must be easy and cheap to avoid. Nudges are not mandates. Putting
fruit at eye level counts as a nudge. Banning junk food does not.'[18]
You will note that a 'nudge' has no negative reinforcement, it
doesn't involve any penalty, economic or otherwise, and it cannot

be mandatory. Yet this theory turned out to be such a powerful influence on so many aspects of human behaviour that Richard Thaler received the 2017 Nobel Prize in Economics for his 'Nudge' theory.[20]

Nudge is based on the simple premise that people, when making decisions quickly (and sometimes even when making decisions with apparent thought), will often choose what is easiest over what is wisest. Supermarkets, for example, have known for ages that where they place items in the store powerfully influences the likelihood of whether they are bought. In supermarkets throughout the world, the ends of aisles are not where shoppers tend to naturally stop, they are seldom the destination. Rather it is a place to be passed by as shoppers U-turn after leaving aisle B (eggs, cakes and bread) on the way to aisle C (canned vegetables, tomatoes and soups), which is where shoppers begin to slow down and look. As a result, the ends of the aisles are where sale items and other special offers are typically placed, in order to entice shoppers to stop and take a look. In contrast, all of the non-sale and 'premium' items, will be placed in between the aisles at eye or grab level. These items are more likely to be in a shopper's eye-line and they are therefore nudged towards a purchase. Crucially, it doesn't matter whether the item at eye or grab level is healthy or not. The shopper will more likely (but clearly not always) buy the item, whether or not they had any idea of or a position on the obesity problem. As many of you would have undoubtedly personally experienced, major soft-drink manufacturers will typically provide their own branded refrigerated units to smaller corner shops or to takeaway outlets, which they will then stock with some of their products. I was in a local fish and chip takeaway one day and noted just such a branded fridge. When I remarked upon this to the proprietor, he gave a very interesting response. Apparently, while he was free to display whatever he wanted in the fridge, he was mandated by the company to place their brand of products at eye or grab level, even within their clearly and colourfully liveried fridge. They, of course, know the science, and are acting to increase the likelihood of you purchasing their brand of beverage.

Not all nudges that exist around us were placed there knowingly. Take the size of our tableware, for instance. Plates have become bigger over the years, largely because of fashion. Most sit-down restaurants now pile the food artistically in the centre of an enormous dish with sauce dotted about wildly in the style of Jackson Pollack (never enough sauce for my liking in these gastro-places), and serve wine in a fishbowl-sized glass. This is fine in a restaurant where food is plated up and served to you. However, what this has meant is that the size of our domestic plates has mirrored this increase, because why would we not, entirely reasonably, want to replicate the restaurant experience in our own kitchens? But at home, we serve ourselves, and people have been shown to consistently consume more food and drink when using larger tableware or glasses. Studies suggest that if reductions in exposure to larger-sized food portions, packages and tableware could be achieved, this could reduce daily energy consumption, based on a UK diet, by between 144 and 228 calories per person.[20] A colleague of mine from the University of Cambridge, Prof. Dame Theresa Marteau ('Dame', for you non-UK readers, is the female equivalent of 'Sir'; and yes I do think that 'Dame' is a pretty lame equivalent for 'Sir' and that in this day and age, the UK really needs to sort this out) conducted a study on the role that wine-glass size played on our wine-purchasing behaviour in a restaurant/bar scenario. In the UK, there is a legal measure for what volume constitutes a 'glass' of wine, which is 175ml. What Theresa did at one of the local Cambridge watering holes was to, on a two-weekly basis over 16 weeks, provide them with different-sized wine glasses. So during a given two-week period, the establishment may have had only small (250ml), medium (300ml) or large (370ml) wine glasses, but the volume of wine poured per glass, irrespective of glass size, remained the same. What Theresa found was that during the weeks where the large (370ml) glasses were in play, 10 per cent more wine was sold by the glass, whereas there was no differences in the bottles of wine sold.[21] If you think about it, it does make sense. A bottle of wine is bought to be shared (typically), and sits on the table, so you can see how much is being drunk. It is therefore a considered decision to purchase a second (or third, or fourth) bottle. However, because humans are notoriously bad at judging volumes in different-sized containers, even when the volumes are a standardised 175ml, the larger glasses had clearly influenced the perceived amount of wine drunk and hence purchased. This same phenomenon is going to be true with plate sizes and the amount of food being served, except there is no standardised amount of food! Anecdotally, I have noticed, for instance, that when I go to a buffet style 'all you can eat' restaurant, the plates they provide tend to be smaller than at a restaurant where food is served for the opposite reason, so you think you are eating more food than you actually are.

So I do think there are some lessons to be learned here. I am not suggesting that everyone throws out their lovely wedding china. But try to be aware of portion sizes if you are the one cooking and/ or serving the food. Also, rather than bringing the pot of stew or chilli or curry and putting it on the dinner table where, without even thinking about it, you can serve yourself some more – leave the pot on the stove. You can still serve yourself more, but you will be making a considered decision to walk to the stove to get more food. When you are shopping for food, realise that 'nudge' is being used by companies all the time, to manipulate you into behaving a certain way, into making certain purchasing decisions. Once you understand how it works, you can try to recognise marketing tricks and avoid bad food and health decisions. I realise that this is far easier said than done, given that companies pay good money to 'nudge' you into all manner of purchasing decisions. But taking steps to make more considered purchases or choices would be a good start.

'YOU CAN'T OUTRUN A BAD DIET'

'Hey, what about exercise?' I hear all you gym bunnies and Insta #fitspo folks asking.

From a personal perspective, I don't happen to be a gym type of person. That's not to say that I am a slug; I am not. Rather, my exercise of choice is road cycling, all of which, sadly these days, is confined to my commute to and from work. I do however, log 14 miles each way, door to door. Throw in the days I have to teach or have meetings in town or at college, and I easily average over 30 miles a day on my bike. I have one of those heart monitor/GPS devices, and it estimates that I expend around 900–1,000 calories a day on my bike, which is, by any measure, quite a lot. Yet, I have a wobbly tummy and a BMI of 26. My wife always wonders, with equal frustration and amazement, why I am not as skinny as a rake. 'A good doer' she calls me, which is a term referring to a horse that does well on its feed and is not difficult to keep 'in condition'. I always wonder what size I would be if I didn't cycle!

You can't outrun a bad diet, so goes the saying. Is that true? There is plenty of evidence that increasing physical activity in and of itself, without considering the food-intake side of the equation, is not an effective way of shedding the pounds.[22] It is, after all, the second law of thermodynamics: you have to burn more than you eat to lose weight. A major problem when you exercise is that you get hungry and you need to refuel. Like judging volumes of wine in different glass sizes, people are also notoriously bad at estimating how many calories were burnt during a given workout, and equally bad at estimating how many calories are in a given portion of food. It also doesn't help that the heart monitor/GPS device-type things are not particularly accurate in measuring calorie expenditure. So what happens is that some people tend to overcompensate in refuelling after a bout of exercise, and end up eating more calories than they actually expended. While the number of additional calories eaten by these 'compensators' varies widely, making it difficult to provide a single meaningful number, experiments show that they have a higher preference for high-fat sweet foods.[23] In my situation, I don't think I'm overcompensating because I've been weight stable for the past seven years, so I'm clearly eating as much as I am burning while on my bike. But a less generous interpretation of the data would be that I've been unable to lose any weight over the past seven years in spite of the distance I cycle per day.

There are people out there, however, who can 'outrun a bad diet'. They are elite endurance athletes. UK long-distance runner Sir Mo Farah, for instance, has to eat nearly 4,000 calories a day when in training, and yet he is my height and weighs nearly 20kg less than I do! Tour de France cyclists burn through an average of 5,000 calories per stage of the 21-stage race! The cyclists actually lose weight during the Tour because they actually don't have enough time in any given 24-hour period to replenish all of the calories they have expended. A typical male elite cross-country skier who, unlike cyclists and runners, uses both arms and legs in their sport, must eat nearly 8,000 calories a day. American swimmer Michael Phelps was famously reported to eat nearly 12,000 calories a day during his training for the 2008 Beijing Olympics.[24] His typical diet, which was detailed with almost envious glee by multiple media outlets, included a breakfast of three fried-egg sandwiches, a five-egg omelette, three pieces of French toast and three pancakes. Lunch was typically a pound of pasta and two sandwiches. For dinner, he would eat an entire large pizza and a pound of pasta. Whether or not that actually adds up to 12,000 calories, I'm not so sure. Bottom line is, you CAN outrun a bad diet. It's just that most of us don't run, cycle, ski or swim for long enough to do it!

The evidence for exercise helping to maintain weight after you've lost it, however, is far stronger.[25] It appears that between 200 and 300 minutes of moderate-intensity exercise per week, equating to between 1,200 and 2,000 calories expended, is probably necessary to enhance long-term weight loss and minimise weight regain following weight loss.[26] Also, remember that there is a benefit to sometimes exercising in a relatively 'fasted' state. The fuel that our bodies will preferentially use during exercise are our carbohydrate stores, which include 100 calories of glucose circulating in the blood, and about 1,900 calories of glycogen stored in your liver and muscles; probably a couple of days' worth. As your carbohydrate stores begin to go down, you will begin to burn fat. So if you start your exercise with lower carbohydrate stores on board, your body will begin to burn fat faster. Exercising in the morning before breakfast, for example, could be beneficial for this reason. But this is something to do periodically, rather than constantly, and you will definitely still want to carbo-load before the big race to maximise your performance!

Critically though, exercise is good for you, *independent* of any weight loss. Regular exercise lowers all-cause mortality and can prevent the onset of obesity, type 2 diabetes, hypertension and cardiovascular disease.[27] So everybody who is able should be encouraged to exercise or be physically active, regardless of the weight loss achieved or not achieved.

WHAT IS THE RIGHT DIET FOR YOU?

So is there a right diet for you? There probably is, although the first thing you have to know is why you are looking to change you eating habits, which is, after all, what 'going on a diet' means. Are you trying to lose weight? Are you trying to get healthier? Do you have heart problems or issues with high blood pressure? Each of us will have different biological endpoints we are trying to reach; thus, each will require subtly different approaches and will take different lengths of time to achieve. It is also likely to be different for everyone because of our own personal mix of genes. You have to understand your own feeding behaviour, you have to be honest with your own foibles and weaknesses, and you have to recognise that it is not going to be easy. And finally, remember that a diet only works, only has its effects, while you are actually on the diet.

A question many people ask is whether there is an optimal 'weight per month' to lose, to maximise your chances of keeping the weight off. The truth is, there is no good data available to con-clusively answer this question. However, losing a large amount of weight in a short period of time will clearly require extreme caloric restriction, which, while achievable in the short term, is very un-likely, for most people, to be maintained over a period of months and years. Common sense tells us that a more moderate reduction of calories will be easier to maintain over a longer period of time. The most important message to take away from this chapter is that the 'right diet' for you is one that works for you and suits your lifestyle, otherwise you are not going to be able to keep it up.

CHAPTER 12

The perfect diet written in your genes

I was on a family hiking holiday in the north of England in the summer of 2016. We were in Yorkshire (of pudding fame) and staying in the little coastal town of Staithes. The weather, unusually for a summer in Yorkshire, was 'Goldilocks' good, so not too hot and not too cold, just enough sun and just enough cloud; perfect outdoor walking conditions. Then in the evenings, after a meal (sometimes even including Yorkshire pudding) and a pint of beer in the pub, we would sit down to watch coverage of the Rio Olympics, which was going on at the time. All in all, it was a fabulous holiday.

I am an avid cyclist, so one of my favourite events to watch was the cycling. Not the road cycling, as I prefer the strategy and masochism of the longer multi-stage races such as the Tour de France; but the crazy explosiveness of track cycling. If you've never watched a bunch of adults going round a polished wooden track on two wheels at ridiculous speeds, I can highly recommend it. The competitors, all of whom have thighs with larger circumferences than the waists of most models, go only one way round a track with crazy banking, on bikes that only have one single enormous gear, with no freewheel and no brakes! It is a sport that the UK particularly excels at. We even have our own 'golden couple' of track cycling, Jason Kenny and Laura Trott, who were at the time engaged to be married (and are now actually married). Between the two of them, they managed to pick up five gold medals in Rio (three for Jason and two for Laura; they have nine gold medals in total, if you included the 2012 London Olympics)! On this particular evening of competition, Laura had already completed all of her events and she was cheering Jason on to winning his third and final gold medal. As the crowd, and we in our small Yorkshire hotel room, roared Jason across the finish-line, Laura tweeted: 'Arghhhh!!!!!! I love him to bits. Our kids have to get some of these genes right?'

For my sins, I occasionally write for a major UK tabloid newspaper. I thought long and hard about it before working with them, particularly as I disagree with their political leanings and the vast majority of their headlines. However, because what I write appears in their Health pages, and I have control over the final 'copy' that appears in print and online, I am comfortable using the platform to put out sensible science messages in an attempt to educate. As a consequence, the health journalist of this particular tabloid paper had me on 'speed dial'. Not 30 minutes after Jason won and gave Laura a big hug and a kiss, my phone buzzed. My wife looked at me: *Who is calling you at this time of the evening?*

I swiped right to answer.

'Giles? This is Doris from the health desk [I have changed her name to protect the innocent]. Were you watching the cycling? Do you think you could put together a few hundred words discussing the likelihood of Jason's and Laura's kids turning out to be Olympians?'

'Excuse me?! Ummm, I'm on holiday at the moment . . .'

'We'll provide you with a ghostwriter. This will be a great piece!'

Doris wasn't kidding and she was insistent.

But then I cogitated about it a bit more, and it did seem like a great opportunity to discuss complex genetics in some depth (relatively speaking). Unlike the colour of Mendel's peas, there clearly wasn't going to be a single gene that determined whether or not someone became an 'Olympic track cyclist'. Rather, it would be down to an optimum mixture of a number of relevant traits, such as aerobic capacity, muscle fibre type, pain threshold, ability to focus, responsiveness to training, to name a few, each of which would be influenced by their own repertoire of many genes. There would also be the important role of the environment. For instance, surely being brought up in a household with two multiple-gold-medal-winning cyclists would also have a powerful influence on their children? Surely the quality of their diets and level of physical activity would be far above the norm? Anyway, the opportunity did seem too good to pass up, so I agreed.

I put the article together, with the help of the ghostwriter, in 48 hours, and it, surprisingly, generated an enormous amount of media interest. In fact, we were still in the middle of our holiday when the piece was published, and I ended up being interviewed live for the main UK satellite news channel, by FaceTime on my phone, from the top of a hill where I had miraculously found some transient 4G coverage. I'm sure it made for gripping television ... my wife found it amusing at any rate. Much of the interest stemmed from the fascination of being able to predict the future, in particular predicting our own futures based on our genes.

THE GENETIC CRYSTAL BALL

Would you pay £249 to find out whether you are genetically predisposed to gaining weight? Or if you're likely to develop high blood pressure if you eat too much salt? Or to become a supertaster? Or if you are better suited to a high-protein diet? That's certainly the hope behind the 'personalised' gene tests now available from companies such as 23andMe, Nutrigenomix and DNAFit. They not only claim their tests can identify genes related to diseases including dementia and obesity, but also predict how you might respond to specific diets, such as low salt, low caffeine or high fat. By using this information, you can then exercise more effectively, lose weight and stay healthy; that is their pitch.[1]

The idea of peering into a genetic crystal ball to predict your future self, or how you might respond to specific treatments and diets should, in principle, be possible. After all, your genes shape who you are and how you respond to the environment. A couple of weeks after the Jason and Laura piece had come out, Doris contacted me again and asked if I was willing to review one of the genetic test products offered by DNAfit? They would pay for me to get the super-duper premium plan, which did indeed cost £249, and then wanted my opinion of the results and their interpretation. From the perspective of intellectual curiosity, it seemed like yet another opportunity too good to miss, so I agreed.

INFORMATION TO HELP ME ACHIEVE MY GENETIC POTENTIAL?

A few days later, a package arrived in my pigeonhole at work. When I brought it back to my office and opened it up, I found a DNAfit-branded cardboard box about the size of an airport paperback novel. The DNAfit strapline, which was found on its logo, was 'Achieve your genetic potential'. On one end of the box was a little 'pull me' tab attached to a drawer. As I tugged at it to see what was in the box, another drawer on the other end of the box, through some unseen mechanism, unexpectedly slid open smoothly and simultaneously. It was all very slick and very swish. I mean, the engineering and design that went into just the box itself was a sight to behold.. In one of the drawers was everything I needed to collect my DNA sample and in the other was the bar-coded paperwork where I had to initial here, here and here, and then sign my life away. I followed the instructions to take a cheek swab, and then put it into the provided container with what I assumed to be some type of preservation solution. I placed everything into the pre-paid, self-addressed and barcoded packaging, and as easy as 1-2-3, my DNA sample was winging its way to DNAfit. Then in a little under two weeks, I received an email containing a clickable link to access and download my results.

The 'premium' option from DNAfit, which is what I plumped for, meant that both my diet and my fitness 'genetic profiles' had been assessed, so I received three different files; a poster summarising the results, one with my detailed fitness results and one with my diet results. Each of the very glossy detailed reports began with a simple genetics primer, some Ts & Cs stating that the information provided was not intended to be a diagnosis, followed by, while not in name, something which certainly looked and smelt like a diagnosis.

Let's start with my fitness results. In total, DNAfit tested 21 different genetic variations, and from there made conclusions about four different 'fitness traits'; my power versus endurance profile, my aerobic potential, my recovery speed and my risk of injury. For instance, illustrated to me using a crazy shape in two different shades of green, my 'power response' was 51.2 per cent as compared to my endurance response which was 48.8 per cent. These appeared to be very specific numbers indeed. They then elaborated:

'Your assessment has determined that your genetic profile is almost equally balanced between power and endurance activities, based on variations in your genes. In your training mix power and endurance activities to benefit from your intermediate profile.'

My aerobic potential, speed of recovery and risk of injury were all confidently predicted to be 'medium'. My reading of these results? I appear to be boringly 'average'.

OK, and how about my personalised diet profile based on my genes? Surely this is why all of you have stuck with this book to Chapter 12, with undoubtedly bated breath? Well, DNAfit tested 25 different genetic variations, 9 of which overlapped with the 'fitness test', and made conclusions about my carbohydrate sensitivity, saturated fat sensitivity, detoxification ability of the liver, antioxidant need, omega-3 need, vitamin B and D requirements, salt, alcohol and caffeine sensitivity, lactose intolerance and predisposition to coeliac disease. Some highlights included, based on my liver's 'detoxification ability', advising me to limit my consumption of grilled or smoked meat to 1–2 servings per week; that I had a raised requirement for B vitamins, in particular B6 and B12; and that I had raised salt sensitivity. Taking all of this information into account, DNAfit assures me that my optimal diet should be a Mediterranean diet, as opposed to a low-carb or low-fat diet.

Keeping in mind that the only personal information that I provided to DNAfit was my age and sex, with no additional anthropometric measurements or even my ethnicity, these were, from both a fitness and diet perspective, pretty extraordinary conclusions to be made. In fact, I'd go so far as to say that the vast majority of predictions provided for me would have been *impossible* to reach based simply on these 37 different genetic variations across both my fitness and diet profiles.

There were two key exceptions, both of which I touched on briefly in Chapter 6. Two of the genes tested were *Alcohol Dehydrogenase 1C (ADH1C)*[2] and *Lactase (LCT)*.[3] I have one copy of a genetic variant of *ADH1C*, which meant that while I could metabolise alcohol, I couldn't drink as much as many of my white Caucasian friends (correctly predicted based upon real world data); and because I lacked the lactase persistence genetic variation at *LCT*, I was lactose intolerant (also correct). Both of these traits, however, are like the colour of Mendel's peas or the severely obese kids lacking leptin,[4] in that they are determined by single genes; these are referred to in genetics as Mendelian traits. As a result, these were accurately predicted by DNAfit. Using the other 35 genetic variations, however, to try and 'predict' some very complex traits is, just simply, fundamentally flawed.

OK, before I get accused of libelling any company or anyone, let me just be crystal clear about what I am saying. First, my criticisms are not levelled only at DNAfit; it just happened to be their product that I was testing out. Rather, all of the companies that attempt to make predictions about complex traits purely based on genetic information are equally flawed. Second, the actual genetic information provided by all of these companies is very likely going to be correct. That is because the technology to determine your precise genetic code is (relatively) cheap and it is robust. Your genetic code is also an empirical measurement, which means that if any vendor gets it wrong, either premeditated or by mistake, they would get in serious trouble for false advertising. In fact, the gene 'diagnostic' sector is very heavily regulated; with specific protocols needing to be followed and ensuring the application of good laboratory practice. For example, even though my lab at the University of Cambridge is perfectly capable of performing genetic tests for research purposes, we are not actually licensed to provide any genetic diagnoses. Interpreting the results, however, is another thing entirely. Finally, the science quoted and used by DNAfit and other personal genetic testing companies to support their claims and make their 'predictions' is, by and large, respectable and sound. The information would have come from epidemiological studies of varying size and robustness, but all would have been peer-reviewed and published in scientific journals.

These companies are not lying. Rather, they are trying to get the data to do what it was not designed to do; they are misinterpreting the genetic results.

INCONVENIENT TRUTHS

Let's look in more detail at why these types of tests aren't able to make accurate predictions. At the end of Chapter 2, I discussed the fact that there are over a hundred genes that are associated with bodyweight and how one could actually create a 'risk score' for our likelihood of becoming obese.[5] To calculate such a score, consider each genetic variant having a possible score of 2 (homozygous for the risk allele), 1 (heterozygous) or 0 (homozygous for the protective allele). With 100 genes, that is a notional maximum risk score of 200 (100 x 2) and a minimum of 0. When plotted against a large enough population, what we observe is the higher your obesity risk score, the higher your BMI is likely to be (see figure 10). Similar types of risk scores can be produced for most complex

Obesity Risk score directly related to BMI in the population

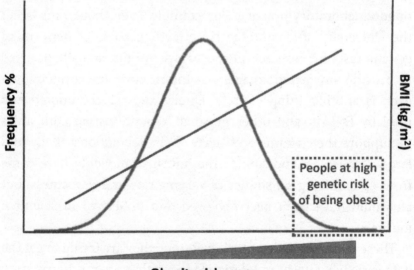

FIGURE 10

diseases and traits. This is, essentially, what these companies are doing; looking at our genes and then comparing it with data that already exists about the rest of the population. The question is, can you take people with an empirically high genetic risk of developing disease – obesity, say – and make a pre-emptive intervention before they become obese? This is, after all, the holy grail of so-called 'precision medicine', where bespoke treatments are designed to fit each individual. The personal genetic testing companies certainly think so.

There are, however, a couple of inconvenient truths that get in the way. Most complex traits (such as height, weight, aerobic capacity or age of puberty) or diseases (such as type 2 diabetes, high blood pressure, rheumatoid arthritis or heart disease) will have a large genetic component that is modulated by the environment. We now know that there are hundreds of genetic variations that influence each of these traits. For instance, if we consider weight as an exemplar, more than a hundred genes had to be studied in hundreds of thousands of individuals in order to show the relationship with BMI.[6] There are rare types of severe obesity, such as those seen in the children with no leptin,[7] that are the result of catastrophic mutations in single genes. This is not the situation for the vast majority of us with 'common' obesity, where there is no one 'obese' gene. Instead, each of us will have our own personal mix of the more than 100 obesity risk vs protective variants. None of the genetic companies, however, test more than a small handful of genes per given trait, including for bodyweight. DNAfit, for example, only test between one to seven genes for each characteristic they are claiming to predict. By examining only a few of the hundreds of known variants, they are already massively reducing the predictive power of the risk score. Inconvenient truth Number 1.

POPULATION RISK VERSUS INDIVIDUAL PREDICTION

It is, however, the second inconvenient truth that presents the real problem. Even if all of the known variations for each trait or characteristic were taken into account, it would make very little measurable difference in the ability of the genetic testing companies to make the predictions they are claiming. Why? Because they are fundamentally misunderstanding the difference between population-level risk and individual diagnosis or prediction. What exactly do I mean by this?

In addition to running a research group at the University of Cambridge, I also do some undergraduate teaching. In particular, I teach a few lectures in biochemistry '101' (mysteriously called 'Molecules In Medical Science' or MIMS) to the first-year pre-clinical medical and veterinary students; I am, in fact, the first lecturer that these students see as they begin their journey as Cambridge students (I know, I know, what did they do to deserve that?) Those of you (myself included) who had the fortune of sitting through first-year biochemistry will recall the rote memorisation of dozens of different biochemical pathways, such as glycolysis or the Krebs cycle, only to have them evaporate from the mind almost immediately after disgorging them on to an exam paper. In an effort to combat this dreadful waste of glucose by the brain, the department has structured the course around disease themes, with the first term focusing on diabetes and obesity, and the second term on cancer. These then formed an architecture on which to place basic biochemical principles into a clinical perspective. In the last lecture of term, though, I leave the curriculum and give the students a talk on the genetics of obesity, not unlike what I've covered in the first few chapters of this book. When I get to the point about risk versus prediction,

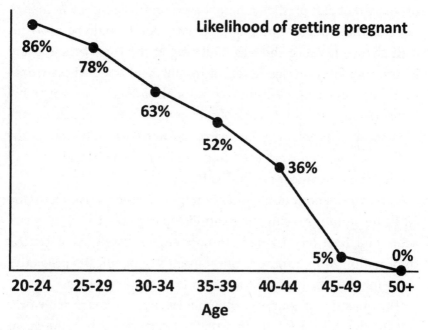

Likelihood of getting pregnant

86%

78%

63%

52%

36%

5%

0%

20-24   25-29   30-34   35-39   40-44   45-49   50+

Age

FIGURE 11

this is the analogy I use to try and illustrate the point.

Let us consider the likelihood of getting pregnant. To the mostly eighteen-year-old first-year undergraduate students to whom I am trying to make the point, it is clearly more of a 'risk', but you get my drift. It is very well known that younger women are more fertile and are therefore more likely to get pregnant than someone older. The graph above illustrates this point, with twenty-to twenty-four-year-old women having an 86 per cent chance, when trying to get pregnant, of actually getting pregnant.[8] This decreases as women get older, till the menopause hits post-fifty, and the likelihood drops to 0 per cent. Given the number of women who have ever been pregnant (a whole lot), plus everything we know about the biology of reproduction, you would imagine the graph to be extremely robust. However, while the likelihood of a woman between the ages of thirty and thirty-four years getting pregnant is 63 per cent, could you take a random thirty-four-year-old woman off the street and predict, simply based on this graph, whether or not she would become pregnant? Clearly not. It could be a 100 per cent chance because she was ovulating at the time, or she could be infertile for a myriad different reasons and the chances would then be 0 per cent. Without additional biological or hormonal information, you simply cannot take population-level data on the likelihood of pregnancy, no matter how robust and how many millions of women were used to generate the graph, and use it to predict the outcome for an individual.

The same analogy holds true for population-level risk scores. So while the graph showing the relationship between the obesity risk score and BMI has, by definition, been generated using genetic information from hundreds of thousands of people, its predictive value for an individual is little better than flipping a coin.

The question of course is why? Given that our genes determine our biology, why am I arguing that we can't use it to predict our health or behaviour? The answer has to do with how much of our genetic code we are actually even looking at and our ability, or more accurately our inability, to effectively 'measure' the environment.

WHAT MAKES US DIFFERENT?

Greater that 99 per cent of the genome is the same in all humans, it is what defines us as human. However, what makes us all different lies in the 0.01 per cent of our DNA, around 30 million base-pairs, that varies between us all. So there we have our first problem; the risk scores are generated from only a minuscule proportion of the DNA that make us different, and an even smaller proportion of our total amount of genetic material. The obesity risk score that I've discussed, for instance, is generated from around just 100 different genetic variations. That is 100 out of 3 billion or 0.00000003 per cent of the genome.

The genetic variations that are associated with disease are also, by and large, the most common ones. These common variants are placed on chips so that up to 3 million can be screened in any given individual at the same time, making it easy to scale up and study millions of variations at a population level. It has proven to be a very powerful technology indeed, allowing scientists to reveal the genetic architecture of complex traits and diseases. However, in addition to these 'known knowns', there are also likely to be 'unknown unknowns', or genetic variations that are rare or 'private' to individual families, that would also play a significant role in disease. Because they are rare or unknown, they can't be easily screened. The only way to do that would be to perform whole genome sequencing on a large number of people. That is beginning to happen now, but is going to take time, a lot of money and the ability to analyse and interpret such an enormous amount of data. The bottom line is, while those 100 variations used to generate the obesity risk score do indeed subtly influence BMI, we just don't know enough, yet, about how these individual variations interact with themselves, let alone with all the rest of the genes and regulatory elements.

MEASURING THE ENVIRONMENT

The two essential ingredients to obtaining meaningful genetic associations on a population level are power (the number of individuals studied, preferably in the tens to hundreds of thousands; here, bigger is undoubtedly better) and an unambiguous and empirical measure or characteristic. When I say empirical, I mean a measure that does not rely on anyone's memory or opinion. So BMI, waist-to-hip ratio or height, for example, are all very easy to obtain, requiring only a set of bathroom scales and a measuring tape, and yet informative. They can all change over time of course, but at any given moment, they do not lie and they are what they are. Then there are slightly more complicated measures such as blood pressure, blood glucose and insulin levels, cholesterol levels and body-fat percentage. These are all unambiguous and empirical measures, but obtaining them requires specialised equipment and/or medically qualified personnel. That being said, they are still relatively easy to collect on a population level.

But then we get to behaviours and characteristics, which on the surface seem very straightforward, but are actually incredibly difficult to measure accurately, particularly in large numbers of people. Measurement of feeding behaviour and energy expenditure – so both sides of the energy-balance equation – most certainly falls into this category.

WHAT AND HOW MUCH WE EAT

Feeding behaviour, broadly speaking, encompasses what and how much you eat. Aspects of feeding behaviour are measurable in small numbers of people within a laboratory setting, but suffers from the perennial conundrum that by studying a behaviour you invariably change the behaviour. So imagine you sign up for a study, and when you arrive on the day and step into the lab, someone produces some food and tells you to 'eat naturally'. Except for young children, this is nearly impossible to do. Adults get self-conscious, they begin to imagine what is being measured . . . *is it the amount of food I am eating? I don't want to look like a glutton* . . . What is possible to measure in this controlled setting is food 'choice', such as the chicken korma and Eton mess study looking into fat and sugar preference that I described in Chapter 2.[9] These types of studies, however, are very difficult to scale up even to hundreds of people, let alone the tens of thousands of people required for population-level studies.

What and how much people eat can be measured at the population level, but it is notoriously difficult to do so accurately. The current 'state of the art' still involves food diaries and questionnaires, which of course aren't state of any art at all. If I asked you what you ate for breakfast just a couple of days ago, chances are you'd remember it was a slice of toast with peanut butter, some steel-cut oats in milk with honey and a mug of white coffee. But the moment you are asked how much you ate of everything, it becomes very tricky. How much butter and peanut butter did you actually spread on the toast? How much porridge, milk and honey actually went into the bowl? How much milk went into your coffee? Now imagine doing that for a meal you had two weeks ago, and you begin to see how such data is entirely at the mercy of opinion and memory.

HOW MUCH WE HAVE BURNT

Energy expenditure, broadly speaking, encompasses three components; basal metabolic rate, diet-induced thermogenesis and physical activity. Your metabolic rate is the energy used to keep your entire body functioning while you are at rest and accounts for about 60 per cent of total energy burnt; diet-induced thermogenesis, which accounts for 10 per cent of expenditure is the heat given off when you eat and digest food; and physical activity is self-explanatory and accounts for around 30 per cent of energy expended. The first two components, which account for 70 per cent of energy expenditure, we cannot actually influence; it is largely determined by our body size, with a healthy dose of genetic influence thrown in. Many people might imagine that smaller, more wiry individuals would burn a lot more energy than a slower and larger person. The reality is actually the opposite; the larger the person, the higher the metabolic rate. The analogy I would use here is to compare a Mini Cooper with a Range Rover (other compact cars and large SUVs are available). While a Mini might seem to be very agile compared to the larger vehicle, it clearly has a far lower fuel consumption than a Range Rover. The larger engine and bigger mass to move about demands more fuel. The same is true for humans (and, in fact, all living creatures).

These first two components can be measured very accurately by placing a person in a 'chamber calorimeter', a completely sealed room in which the exact amount of oxygen and carbon dioxide going in and coming out of the room is recorded. This is pretty much the 'gold-standard'. Keeping with the vehicle analogy, we breathe in oxygen as fuel and breathe out carbon dioxide as exhaust, so measuring the ins and outs of this process allows us to indirectly calculate energy expenditure. You have to live in the chamber calorimeter for a few days, during which your metabolic rate can be measured when you are resting, when you are eating and, if there is a stationary bike in the room, when you are exercising. But as you might imagine, such rooms are technologically very complex, and as such there are only a handful in the UK for instance. So this method, although invaluable in a clinical or research setting, cannot be realistically scaled up to a population level. Instead, when measuring energy expenditure beyond a handful of individuals, portable hoods that can be placed over one's head are used instead. This follows the same principle of measuring oxygen used and carbon dioxide produced, but is less accurate because the hood is not airtight and measurements are taken over a far shorter period of time; typically around 30 minutes. Even so, this technique remains time-consuming and labour-intensive and scaling up beyond a few thousand people is very challenging.

The 30 per cent of energy expended that is encompassed by physical activity is the only component we can actively influence. It is easier to measure because of the proliferation of wearable fitness monitors that have flooded the market. These range from technically advanced accelerometers, with inbuilt heart-rate monitors and gyroscopes that can tell if you are standing, sitting or lying down, to simple pedometers that count the number of steps you might accumulate in a day, and everything in between. What is interesting is that while in the short term owning one of these monitors does seem to have a beneficial effect in terms of activity and weight loss, sadly these effects disappear in the long term, presumably when we begin to ignore or tire of what used to be the exciting new toy on our wrists.[10]

Currently, most of the genes linked to BMI produce proteins that function in the brain, many of which, including components of the melanocortin pathway such as POMC and MC4R, regulate food intake.[11] To date, however, there are no genes that have been convincingly linked to metabolism and energy expenditure. Does that mean that differences in metabolic rate don't influence BMI? Absolutely not. Food-intake data is simply easier to collect from large numbers of people. So even though food diaries and questionnaires are far from perfect, you can mitigate against the imperfect data to a degree with a large enough dataset. The most likely explanation for the lack of energy expenditure genes associated with BMI is the difficulty of measuring it accurately in a large enough population.

So there we have our second problem. Until we find better and more accurate ways of measuring the environment, such as what people eat and the amount of energy they burn, the predictions based on just a genetic risk score being claimed by the various personal gene testing companies are simply not (yet) possible. In fact, I have spoken to quite a few people who have taken these tests. Almost universally, the predictions, with small variations, are that everyone needs to eat more healthily, maybe Mediterranean-style, and everyone needs to move a little bit more, with a balance of aerobic and resistance training. These tests say that they are giving personalised advice, but end up giving common-sense 'healthy-living' advice, which I could have given to you for free.

THE DAWN OF NUTRIGENOMICS?

Are there going to be genetic influences on our preference for protein, fat (me), carbs or sugar? Yes. Will our genes play a role in whether we will respond to a high-protein, versus a low-carb high-fat, versus a low-GI, versus a Mediterranean diet? Undoubtedly. Are there genes involved in whether or not we eat when we are stressed, and whether or not we live to eat (me) or eat to live (not me)? One hundred per cent. Are there genes that make it more difficult for someone to lose weight and keep it off than someone else; genes that make some of us feel hungrier than others; genes that simply make some of us more efficient with calories than others? Yes, yes and yes.

As I have mentioned, every single one of our traits, behaviours, characteristics and tendencies will have a genetic component. The trick is to find out what genes are involved, how they are involved and how large a role they play. For instance, the 100 BMI genes probably cover the full ambit above. So just simply knowing that someone has a higher than average genetic risk for being obese, such as the 'Constant Cravers' in Chapter 11, doesn't mean you can predict if they will become obese, or pinpoint the exact reasons why they have become obese. Although the genetic risk score is an empirical number, each individual's mix of genetic variations that lead to the score will be different. In other words, we will all have our own unique reasons that lead us to eat more or less or an average amount.

Do I think that at some point in the future we will be able to ac-tually do what the personal genetic testing companies are currently (mistakenly) claiming they can do? Do I believe there is a future for this field of 'nutrigenomics'? Do I believe that 'the perfect diet' for each of us is somewhere to be found in our genes? Yes, I do. But until we are able to be more sophisticated in our analysis of genetic information and couple it to a far better capability of measuring our environment, that time is not now.

CAN WE CHANGE OUR GENES?

As a geneticist working in obesity, I am often asked if we can change our genes to fix our obesity. Given the advances over the past few years in the field of 'gene editing', the question is not as far-fetched as you might imagine. While we have possessed the ability to modify DNA for a few decades now, it was always limited by the organisms we could actually genetically engineer (mostly mice and a few plants) and the areas in the genome that were accessible. The development of CRISPR-Cas9, which is short for **C**lustered **R**egularly **I**nterspaced **S**hort **P**alindromic **R**epeats and CRISPR-**as**sociated protein **9**, however, has now given scientists the ability to change the DNA of any organism or cell, and at pretty much any location in the genome.[12] Developed from a naturally occurring bacterial defence mechanism, CRISPR-Cas9 acts simultaneously as both molecular scalpel and tweezers, allowing very precise editing of the genome to occur. It is most certainly 'now technology' in that it is in wide use in laboratories throughout the world; although most scientists, myself included, use it to edit the DNA of cells and of animal models, purely for the purposes of research.

But the great excitement and interest is to use it in the prevention and treatment of human diseases. It is already being used, for example, in the treatment of certain types of cancer. This is done by taking immune cells out of a patient with cancer, modifying them using gene editing to give them the ability to recognise a specific protein on cancer cells, after which they are infused back into the patient. This process, in effect, 'weaponises' the immune cells and programmes them to attack the cancer cells. This approach, however, does not result in any heritable changes. Once the immune cells have done their job, the body gets rid of them. Ethical concerns arise when we begin to discuss altering the human genome in a way that can be passed on to the next generation, which means editing egg or sperm cells or embryos themselves. While it is technically possible to do it now, there is the big question of safety. How sure can we be that by changing one bit of the genome, we don't change something else, for instance? Also, while removing a debilitating genetic condition so that it doesn't blight a family ever again would seem a no-brainer, what happens when people want to begin to change their eye colour, their hair colour or, heaven forbid, their weight? I am not proffering an opinion either way, but this is a discussion that society needs to have, and soon. In the meantime, based on concerns about ethics and safety, editing of egg and sperm cells and embryos is currently illegal in most countries.

The other thing about gene-editing technologies, ethical and safety questions notwithstanding, is that they are currently only able to make single changes to the genome. So it would in theory, for example, be possible to fix the mutation causing leptin deficiency in those kids I told you about back in Chapter 2. However, if you had a high genetic risk for obesity, you would not be able to change fifty or sixty genetic variants, in an attempt to lower your obesity risk score.

HAND OF POKER

Another question I am asked as a geneticist studying obesity is whether I feel I am simply providing obese people with an excuse? With a genetic crutch? It is an interesting question, but one that seems to only be asked about the genetics of a 'behaviour'. So if instead I was studying the genetics of heart disease, or osteoporosis, or arthritis or Alzheimer's or Parkinson's, would people ask me the same question? Would I be giving people suffering from those diseases an excuse as well? What I, and everyone else in the field of obesity genetics, is trying to understand is the biology underlying the problem, because if we don't understand the problem, then we can't fix it.

I always consider our genes to be like a hand of poker. You could get a good hand or you could get a bad hand, and the only people you can blame are your folks. But you can win with a bad hand of poker – it's more difficult, but you can do it – and you can certainly lose with a good hand of poker. So it depends how you play the cards. Using another analogy, I will never ever be able to run as fast as Usain Bolt. A large part of that (it's my excuse and I'm sticking to it) is going to be down to my genes. However, that doesn't mean that if I trained, I wouldn't be able to run faster. Yes, your genes do set limits on what is possible, but for the most part they are not 'deterministic'; rather, your genes give a range of possible outcomes, depending on how they interact with the environment. It's all about trying to reach your genetic potential for any given trait; be it a student at university working hard and trying to reach their genetic potential for intelligence, or an Olympic athlete trying to maximise their genetic potential for physicality or athleticism by eating well and training hard. An obese person, because of the genes they carry, some of which may have been a holdover from the 'feast-famine' environment all those tens of thousands of years on the Serengeti, needs to work harder than others to lose weight and to keep it off. I recall a conversation I had with one of the 'Constant Cravers' I worked with on the *Right Diet* programme. I had told him that he had a high obesity risk score, and that likely played a role in why he found it difficult to lose weight. But I also told him that there was no magic bullet, no magic pill, and he still needed to eat less to lose the weight. What he told me will stick with me to my grave:

'I have been large all my life. I was made fun of as a kid at school. I've been called some very awful things as an adult that I won't repeat. I know there is no magic pill. But now I know that when I am finding it really difficult to say no to food, when the weight just won't go off, that I am NOT a bad person. It is difficult because I am fighting my genes. That makes a huge difference in motivation for me. Thank you so much for helping me.'

Obese people are not lazy, or weak, or morally bereft; they are most certainly not bad. They are fighting their genes, they are struggling against their biology. Until we in society understand that, until we are able to remove the stigma from being obese, we are never, ever, going to be able to fix the problem.

'Yeo truths'

At the outset, I said that this wasn't meant to be a diet book. In fact, I actually said I was writing an 'anti-diet' book. For most of history, the word 'diet' had a positive connotation. It came from the Greek *diaita*, meaning 'a way of life', which conjures such a beautiful image, for food is indeed a way of life.

I am clearly not anti-'way-of-life'.

Somewhere along the way however, 'diet' has become a toxic word, full of judgement. It has infused fear into our relationship with food. It has infused fear of food into us. A case in point is Gwyneth Paltrow's controversial lifestyle brand GOOP, which offered readers tips on how to achieve their 'leanest liveable weight'. Just say that out loud to yourself, and you begin to realise what a fine and dangerous line that is. If that doesn't illustrate, with crystal clarity, the infusion of fear into food, I don't know what else will.

I am anti-'fear-of-food'.

Do we have a problem with our food environment that we need to fix? Are obesity and other diet-related illnesses killing us? Of course. I am not blind to these problems; my day job is studying obesity after all. But the current tenor of the conversation . . . nay, that is a gross understatement . . . the current shouting and frothing surrounding diets is not helping and is not going to help anyone. For many people, too many, diets have become tribal, almost religious. They believe that keto or plant-based or grain-free or intermittent fasting or Mediterranean is THE right diet. They are on it, it works for them, so it must work for everyone else. They then get personally offended and push back when someone else says they find it difficult, or that it isn't effective for them, or it doesn't suit them; almost like it is an attack on themselves. Why? I guess in a world where so many things are out of control, your diet is something you can control. I am all for taking control of your diet, but do it positively and not out of fear. Just understand that there is no one 'right' diet for everyone. I know it seems like a cliché, but dude, everyone IS different. Everyone behaves differently around food, everyone has a different relationship with food. Consequently everyone will have a different strategy that will work best for them if and when they need to lose weight and to keep it off. You just need to iterate towards a strategy that works for you.

At the early stages of putting this book together, when I was meeting with different publishers, everyone asked *What is the take-home message? Where is your advice to your readers?*

To be frank, I initially pushed back on those questions. This was not a diet book, so I was not going to give any dietary advice, and that was that. But as I've gone through the (sometimes glacially slow) process of writing, I gradually realised that there are some universal truths, some 'Yeo truths' even, that have emerged that are probably worth sharing.

YEO TRUTH #1
IT AIN'T S'POSED TO BE EASY

If anyone tries to sell you an effortless way to lose weight, where you can slim down by paying someone money, where you eat something and it will make you shrink, it is NOT true. They are lying to you. If anyone tries to tell you that magic diet X is magically magic and will work for everyone, as long as it is done correctly, they are lying. In this book, I haven't tried to sugar-coat anything, I haven't tried to sell you a dodgy second-hand car, where the best tyre is on the spare wheel in the trunk/boot. Weight loss is difficult, it is hard. Our biology makes it hard. So you shouldn't feel bad if it feels hard, because it ain't s'posed to be easy. What you have to do is to chip away at it a little at a time, with a little help from Yeo truths #2–6.

YEO TRUTH #2
EAT A LITTLE LESS OF EVERYTHING

Preach! Ladies and gents, moderation, boring though it is, difficult though it is, is still the answer. So don't demonise and exclude whole food groups (unless medically warranted). Too much of ANYthing is bad (meat, fat, sugar and even carrots), and too little of anything is also bad (including sugar and fat).

YEO TRUTH #3
FOOD THAT TAKES LONGER TO DIGEST
GENERALLY MAKES YOU FEEL FULLER

Food that takes longer to digest will travel farther down the gut and make you feel fuller. Because protein is the most chemically complex of the macronutrients, it takes the longest to digest, which is part of the reason that a calorie of protein will make you feel fuller than a calorie of fat or carbs. So a *moderate* (moderate is critically important here) increase in protein (limiting red and processed meats) can help with weight loss. Remember, any protein will have this effect, not just meat.

Carbs that take longer to digest, such as complex whole grains containing fibre, also travel farther down the gut making you feel fuller. They also release their energy more evenly, which helps you feel less hungry between meals.

YEO TRUTH #4
DON'T BLINDLY COUNT CALORIES

Calorie counting, without taking into account caloric availability, is meaningless. Remember, 100 calories of sugar vs 100 calories of sweetcorn vs 100 calories of corn tortillas.

YEO TRUTH #5
EAT MORE UNSATURATED FATS

Try to eat more unsaturated fats, such as those in olive oil, nuts and fish, and limit saturated fats. Remember that higher consumption of unsaturated fats has been clearly linked with lower mortality; a worthwhile goal, I think you would agree!

YEO TRUTH #6
DON'T FEAR FOOD

You need to not fear food, you need to work with food. Try and understand food better. I hope that in this book I have provided you with information to help you navigate our modern food environment and the inevitable new fads and diets that ebb and flow every year. I hope that by not being hysterical and not over-interpreting data that is out there, this book can be a go-to for those wanting sensible advice. All I'm trying to do is to provide a base-level knowledge, to equip the public with something useful when they go into the supermarket or look into the cupboard for the next meal. Losing weight will always be difficult, particularly in this current environment. I hope I have given you at least some tools with which to sort the wheat (not evil unless you are a coeliac) from the chaff, the sheep from the goats (but please limit red meat) . . . you get the idea.

It has been an honour and a privilege to have been given this opportunity to share my thoughts and musings with you.

Go forth, be sensible, be moderate (and to paraphrase Oscar Wilde) even with moderation.

ACKNOWLEDGEMENTS

OK, I am fully aware that acknowledgements like this always teeter on the edge of reading like a tediously long awards ceremony speech. That being said, seldom is one given the platform to thank the many people that have chaperoned them along the way; so I hope you will indulge me as I grasp the opportunity.

This whole adventure started when a dude named Charlie Brotherstone rang me up soon after I appeared as an expert contributor on *What's the Right Diet for You?*, which went out on the BBC in 2015. Charlie was a literary agent, and given that I had never spoken to any kind of agent before (except for a travel agent . . . but I don't think that counted), I was quite excited. My excitement dimmed quite rapidly, however, when Charlie asked if I had any interest in writing a cookbook. I told him no. I probably had a book lurking around in my mind somewhere, but it almost certainly was NOT a cookbook. Charlie, undeterred, was keen to meet up anyway. One thing led to another and Charlie ended up representing me. He has, over the past few years, somehow managed to coax this book out of my head and into reality.

All the love in the world to my mom Philomena, my dad Peter, and my sisters Gillian and Gwendoline for making me who I am.

Many thanks to my PhD supervisor, Sydney Brenner, for taking a risk by letting me into his lab in Cambridge all those years ago and sparking my curiosity in genetics.

I have spent my entire professional scientific career with my mentor Stephen O'Rahilly, first as a young post-doc and then as a faculty member in his department; all in all, more than 20 years. Thank you for all you have taught me and for giving me the space to grow and to fly.

My life as a scientist would not be complete without my closest colleague, my 'brother from another mother', Tony Coll, with whom I am able to talk about anything and everything. All the gratitude in the world, as well, to the entire crew of super scientists in Bay 2 of the Metabolic Research Labs.

I still don't know what possessed the editor of BBC *Horizon*, Steve Crabtree, to stick his neck out for me and give me my first break in front of the camera as a presenter; but he did, and it has opened new horizons (pun intended) for me, for which I still pinch myself everyday, just to make sure it is real. I will be forever grateful for the opportunities Steve has afforded me. Thanks to Alicky Sussman and Milla Harrison, who gently and patiently navigated me through that first *Horizon* documentary. It is only because of them that I survived the experience, and have been allowed by the BBC to continue!

The biggest of 'shout outs' go to Tristan Quinn, who directed, and Zoe Hunter Gordon who was the researcher on the *Clean Eating* film. My experiences in making the documentary were seminal and crystallized my thoughts for this book.

To Amanda Harris at Seven Dials, Orion, for trusting in me and in this project.

To Sarah Jordan for her help, even as a final-year student who had more important things to worry about, in helping me with invaluable research for this book.

To my son Harry for putting up with me, even as I travelled or locked myself in the office to write.

Finally, to my best friend and the love of my life, Jane. She has made me a better person and a better scientist. She believed I could do anything, even when I wavered. This book would never have happened without her.

ABOUT THE AUTHOR

Giles Yeo is a geneticist with over 20 years' experience dedicated to researching obesity and the brain control of food intake. He obtained his PhD from the University of Cambridge and assisted the pioneering research that uncovered key pathways in how the brain controls food intake. His current research focuses on understanding how these pathways differ from person to person, and the influence of genetics in our relationship with food and eating habits. He is based at the MRC Metabolic Diseases Unit, where he is director of Genomics, and is a fellow and graduate tutor at Wolfson College. Giles also moonlights as science presenter for the BBC.

He lives with his family in a little village with two windmills (one of which mills actual flour), two churches (one deconsecrated) and a pub, just outside Cambridge.

REFERENCES

1. Are your genes to blame when your jeans don't fit?

1. www.oecd.org/health/health-data.htm Accessed 22 May, 2018.
2. www.oecd.org/health/health-data.htm Accessed 22 May, 2018.
3. https://www.cdc.gov/obesity/data/prevalence-maps.html Accessed 22 May, 2018.
4. http://www.pbs.org/independentlens/films/twin-sisters/ Accessed 22 May, 2018.
5. Bailey, R.E., Hatton, T.J. and Inwood, K., 'Health, Height and the Household at the Turn of the 20th Century.' *IZA Discussion Paper* No. 8128 (April 2014).
6. Stunkard, A.J., Foch, T.T. and Hrubec, Z., 'A twin study of human obesity.' *JAMA* 256 (1986);51–4; and Stunkard, A.J., Harris, J.R., Pedersen, N.L. and McClearn, G.E., 'The body-mass index of twins who have been reared apart.' *N Engl J Med* 322 (1990); 1483–87.
7. Schulz, L.O. and Chaudhari, L.S., 'High-Risk Populations: The Pimas of Arizona and Mexico.' *Curr Obes Rep* 4(1) (March 2015); 92–8. doi: 10.1007/s13679-014-0132-9. Review. PMID: 25954599.
8. Neel, J.V., 'Diabetes Mellitus: A "Thrifty" Genotype Rendered Detrimental by "Progress"?' *Am J Hum Genet* 14 (4) (1962); 353–62. PMC 1932342. PMID 13937884.
9. http://www.who.int/gho/ncd/risk_factors/overweight/en/ Accessed 22 May, 2018.

2. It's all in your head

1. Ingalls, A. M., Dickie, M. M. & Snell, G. D., 'Obese, a new mutation in the house mouse.' *J Hered* 41 (1950), 317–18.
2. Hummel, K. P., Dickie, M. M. & Coleman, D. L., 'Diabetes, a new mutation in the mouse.' *Science*: 153 (1966), 1127–28.
3. Coleman, D. L., 'Effects of parabiosis of obese with diabetes and normal mice.' *Diabetologia* 9 (1973), 294–8.
4. Zhang, Y. *et al.*, 'Positional cloning of the mouse obese gene and its human homologue.' *Nature* 372 (1994), 425–32, doi:10.1038/372425a0.
5. Chen, H. *et al.*, 'Evidence that the diabetes gene encodes the leptin receptor: identification of a mutation in the leptin receptor gene in db/db mice.' *Cell* 84 (1996), 491–5.

6. Montague, C. T. *et al.*, 'Congenital leptin deficiency is associated with severe early-onset obesity in humans.' *Nature* 387 (1997), 903–8, doi:10.1038/43185.

7. Farooqi, I. S. *et al.*, 'Effects of recombinant leptin therapy in a child with congenital leptin deficiency.' *N Engl J Med* 341 (1999), 879–84, doi:10.1056/NEJM199909163411204.

8. Heymsfield, S. B. *et al.*, 'Recombinant leptin for weight loss in obese and lean adults: a randomized, controlled, dose-escalation trial.' *JAMA* 282 (1999), 1568–75.

9. Ahima, R. S. *et al.*, 'Role of leptin in the neuroendocrine response to fasting.' *Nature* 382, (1996), 250–52, doi:10.1038/382250a0.

10. Farooqi, I. S. *et al.*, 'Effects of recombinant leptin therapy . . .'

11. For those who are interested, here are some comprehensive reviews on the subject: Bluher, M., 'Adipokines – removing road blocks to obesity and diabetes therapy.' *Mol Metab* 3 (2014), 230–40, doi:10.1016/j.molmet.2014.01.005; Fasshauer, M. & Bluher, M., 'Adipokines in health and disease.' *Trends Pharmacol Sci* 36 (2015), 461–70, doi:10.1016/j.tips.2015.04.014.

12. Aficionados can read reviews that many have written on the topic: Coll, A. P., Farooqi, I. S. & O'Rahilly, S., 'The hormonal control of food intake.' *Cell* 129 (2007), 251–62, doi:10.1016/j.cell.2007.04.001; Cone, R. D., 'Anatomy and regulation of the central melanocortin system.' *Nat Neurosci* 8 (2005), 571–8, doi:10.1038/nn1455; Yeo, G. S. & Heisler, L. K., 'Unraveling the brain regulation of appetite: lessons from genetics.' *Nat Neurosci* 15 (2012), 1343–49, doi:10.1038/nn.3211.

13. Raffan, E. *et al.*, 'A Deletion in the Canine POMC Gene Is Associated with Weight and Appetite in Obesity-Prone Labrador Retriever Dogs.' *Cell Metab* 23 (2016), 893–900, doi:10.1016/j.cmet.2016.04.012.

14. Yeo, G. S. & Heisler, L. K., 'Unraveling the brain regulation of appetite: lessons from genetics.' *Nat Neurosci* 15 (2012), 1343–49, doi:10.1038/nn.3211.

15. Krude, H. *et al.*, 'Severe early-onset obesity, adrenal insufficiency and red hair pigmentation caused by POMC mutations in humans.' *Nat Genet* 19 (1998), 155–7, doi:10.1038/509.

16. Raffan, E. *et al.*, 'A Deletion in the Canine POMC Gene . . .'

17. Yeo, G. S. *et al.*, 'A frameshift mutation in MC4R associated with dominantly inherited human obesity.' *Nat Genet* 20 (1998), 111–12, doi:10.1038/2404.

18. Farooqi, I. S. *et al.*, 'Clinical spectrum of obesity and mutations in the melanocortin 4 receptor gene.' *N Engl J Med* 348, (2003), 1085–95, doi:10.1056/NEJMoa022050.

19. Alharbi, K. K. *et al.*, 'Prevalence and functionality of paucimorphic and private MC4R mutations in a large, unselected European British population, scanned by meltMADGE.' *Hum Mutat* 28 (2007), 294–302, doi:10.1002/humu.20404.

20. Farooqi, I. S. *et al.*, 'Clinical spectrum . . .'

21. van der Klaauw, A. A. *et al.*, 'Divergent effects of central melanocortin signalling on fat and sucrose preference in humans.' *Nat Commun* 7 (2016), 13055, doi:10.1038/ncomms13055.

22. Kim, K. S., Larsen, N., Short, T., Plastow, G. and Rothschild, M. F., 'A missense variant of the porcine melanocortin-4 receptor (MC4R) gene is associated with fatness, growth, and feed intake traits.' *Mamm Genome* 11 (2000), 131–5.

23. Aspiras, A. C., Rohner, N., Martineau, B., Borowsky, R. L. & Tabin, C. J., 'Melanocortin 4 receptor mutations contribute to the adaptation of cavefish to nutrient-poor conditions.' *Proc Natl Acad Sci U S A* 112 (2015), 9668–73, doi:10.1073/pnas.1510802112.

24. Frayling, T. M. *et al.*, 'A common variant in the FTO gene is associated with body mass index and predisposes to childhood and adult obesity.' *Science* 316 (2007), 889–94, doi:10.1126/science.1141634.

25. Locke, A. E. *et al.*, 'Genetic studies of body mass index yield new insights for obesity biology.' *Nature* 518 (2015), 197–206, doi:10.1038/nature14177.

26. Shungin, D. *et al.*, 'New genetic loci link adipose and insulin biology to body fat distribution.' *Nature* 518 (2015), 187–96, doi:10.1038/nature14132.

27. Loos, R. J., 'Genetic determinants of common obesity and their value in prediction.' *Best Pract Res Clin Endocrinol Metab* 26 (2012), 211–26, doi:10.1016/j.beem.2011.11.003.

28. Locke, A. E. *et al.*, 'Genetic studies of body mass index . . .'

3. All calories are equal, but same calories are more equal than others

1. Nestle, M., and Nesheim, M., *Why Calories Count: From Science to Politics*, (University of California Press, 18 April 2012), pp. 189–90. ISBN 978-0-520-26288-1.

2. https://ndb.nal.usda.gov/ndb/ Accessed May 22nd, 2018.

3. Nestle, M. and Nesheim, M., *Why Calories Count . . .*

4. Crockett, R.A., King, S.E., Marteau, T.M., Prevost, A.T., Bignardi, G., Roberts, N.W., Stubbs, B., Hollands, G.J., Jebb, S.A., 'Nutritional labelling for healthier food or non-alcoholic drink purchasing and consumption.' *Cochrane Database Syst Rev* (Feb 27, 2018); 2:CD009315. doi: 10.1002/14651858.CD009315.pub2. Review. PMID: 29482264.

5. www.nobelprize.org/nobel_prizes/medicine/laureates/2017 Accessed 22 May 2018.

6. Zehring, W.A., Wheeler, D.A., Reddy, P., Konopka, R.J., Kyriacou, C.P., Rosbash, M., and Hall, J.C., 'P-element transformation with period locus DNA restores rhythmicity to mutant, arrhythmic Drosophila melanogaster.' *Cell 39* (1984), 369–76; and Bargiello, T.A., Jackson, F.R., and Young, M.W., 'Restoration of circadian behavioural rhythms by gene transfer in Drosophila.' *Nature* 312 (1984), 752–4.

7. Hoyle, N.P., Seinkmane, E., Putker, M., Feeney, K.A., Krogager, T.P., Chesham, J.E., Bray, L.K., Thomas, J.M., Dunn, K., Blaikley, J. and O'Neill, J.S., 'Circadian actin dynamics drive rhythmic fibroblast mobilization during wound healing.' *Sci Transl Med* (Nov 8, 2017); 9(415). pii: eaal2774. doi: 10.1126/scitranslmed.aal2774. PMID: 29118260.

8. Garaulet, M., Gómez-Abellán, P., Alburquerque-Béjar, J.J., Lee, Y.C., Ordovás, J.M., Scheer, F.A., 'Timing of food intake predicts weight loss effectiveness.' *Int J Obes* (Lond., Apr 2013); 37(4):604–11. doi: 10.1038/ijo.2012.229. Epub Jan 29, 2013. Erratum in: *Int J Obes* (Lond., Apr 2013); 37(4):624. PMID: 23357955.

9. Jakubowicz, D., Barnea, M., Wainstein, J. and Froy, O., 'High caloric intake at breakfast vs dinner differentially influences weight loss of overweight and obese women.' *Obesity* (Silver Spring, Dec 2013); 21(12):2504–12. doi: 10.1002/oby.20460. Epub Jul 2, 2013. PMID: 23512957.

10. Baron, K.G., Reid, K.J., Kern, A.S. and Zee, P.C., 'Role of sleep timing in caloric intake and BMI.' *Obesity* (Silver Spring, July, 2011); 19(7):1374–81. doi: 10.1038/oby.2011.100. Epub Apr 28, 2011. PMID: 21527892.

11. Zhang, Y. *et al.*, 'Positional cloning of the mouse obese gene and its human homologue.' *Nature* 372 (1994), 425–32, doi:10.1038/372425a0.
12. Fasshauer, M. and Bluher, M., 'Adipokines in health and disease.' *Trends Pharmacol Sci* 36 (2015), 461–70, doi:10.1016/j.tips.2015.04.014.
13. Vidal-Puig, A., 'Adipose tissue expandability, lipotoxicity and the metabolic syndrome.' *Endocrinol Nutr* (2013); 60 Suppl 1:39–43. PMID: 24490226.
14. Foster, M.T., Shi, H., Softic, S., Kohli, R., Seeley, R.J. and Woods, S.C., 'Transplantation of non-visceral fat to the visceral cavity improves glucose tolerance in mice: investigation of hepatic lipids and insulin sensitivity.' *Diabetologia* (Nov, 2011); 54(11):2890–9. doi: 10.1007/s00125-011-2259-5. Epub Jul 30, 2011. PMID: 21805228.
15. Stolarczyk, E., 'Adipose tissue inflammation in obesity: a metabolic or immune response?' *Curr Opin Pharmacol* (Dec 2017); 37:35–40. doi: 10.1016/j.coph.2017.08.006. Epub Aug 24, 2017. Review. PMID: 28843953.
16. Lotta, L.A., Gulati, P., Day, F.R., Payne, F., Ongen, H., van de Bunt, M., Gaulton, K.J., Eicher, J.D., Sharp, S.J., Luan, J., De Lucia Rolfe, E., Stewart, I.D., Wheeler, E., Willems, S.M., Adams, C., Yaghootkar, H., EPIC-InterAct Consortium; Cambridge FPLD1 Consortium, Forouhi, N.G., Khaw, K.T., Johnson, A.D., Semple, R.K., Frayling, T., Perry, J.R., Dermitzakis, E., McCarthy, M.I., Barroso, I., Wareham, N.J., Savage, D.B., Langenberg, C., O'Rahilly, S. and Scott, R.A., 'Integrative genomic analysis implicates limited peripheral adipose storage capacity in the pathogenesis of human insulin resistance.' *Nat Genet* (Jan 2017); 49(1):17–26. doi: 10.1038/ng.3714. Epub Nov 14, 2016. PMID: 27841877.
17. https://www.nzssd.org.nz/about-diabetes Accessed May 22nd, 2018.
18. Chernev, A., 'The Dieter's Paradox.' *Journal of Consumer Psychology* 21 (2011), 178–83; and Chernev, A. and Gal, D., 'Categorization Effects in Value Judgments: Averaging Bias in Evaluating Combinations of Vices and Virtues.' *Journal of Marketing Research* 47 (2010), 738–47.
19. Forwood, S.E., Ahern, A., Hollands, G.J., Fletcher, P.C. and Marteau, T.M., 'Underestimating calorie content when healthy foods are present: an averaging effect or a reference-dependent anchoring effect?' *PLoS One* (Aug 14, 2013), 8(8):e71475. doi: 10.1371/journal.pone.0071475. eCollection 2013. PMID: 23967216.

4. Should we eat like the Flintstones?

1. Voegtlin, Walter L., *The Stone Age Diet: based on in-depth studies of human ecology and the diet of man*, (Vantage Press, 1975).
2. Cordain, L., *The Paleo Diet Revised: Lose Weight and Get Healthy by Eating the Foods You Were Designed to Eat* (Houghton Mifflin Harcourt, 2010).
3. Cordain, L., Eaton, S.B., Sebastian, A., Mann, N., Lindeberg, S., Watkins, B.A., O'Keefe, J.H. and Brand-Miller, J., 'Origins and evolution of the Western diet: health implications for the 21st century.' *The American Journal of Clinical Nutrition*, Volume 81, Issue 2, (1 February, 2005), pp. 341–54.
4. Cordain, L., *The Paleo Diet Revised: Lose Weight and Get Healthy by Eating the Foods You Were Designed to Eat* (Houghton Mifflin Harcourt, 2010), Preface to the revised edition
5. thepaleodiet.com/the-paleo-diet-premise/ Accessed 5 May 2018.
6. Shewry, P.R., 'Wheat.' *Journal of Experimental Botany*, Volume 60, Issue 6 (1 April 2009), pp. 1537–53, https://doi.org/10.1093/jxb/erp058.

7. Sweeney, M., McCouch, S., 'The complex history of the domestication of rice.' *Ann Bot* (Nov 2007); 100(5):951–7. Epub 2007 Jul 6. Review. PMID: 17617555; and Callaway, E., 'Domestication: The birth of rice.' *Nature* (Oct 30, 2014); 514(7524):S58–9. PMID: 25368889.

8. Ranere, A.J., Piperno, D.R., Holst, I., Dickau, R. and Iriarte, J., 'The cultural and chronological context of early Holocene maize and squash domestication in the Central Balsas River Valley, Mexico.' *Proc Natl Acad Sci U S A* (Mar 31, 2009); 106(13):5014–8. doi: 10.1073/pnas.0812590106. Epub 2009 Mar 23. PMID: 19307573; and Piperno, D.R., Ranere, A.J., Holst, I., Iriarte, J. and Dickau, R., 'Starch grain and phytolith evidence for early ninth millennium B.P. maize from the Central Balsas River Valley, Mexico.' *Proc Natl Acad Sci USA* (Mar 31, 2009); 106(13):5019–24. doi: 10.1073/pnas.0812525106. Epub 2009 Mar 23. PMID: 19307570.

9. Mummert, A., Esche, E., Robinson, J. and Armelagos, G.J., 'Stature and robusticity during the agricultural transition: evidence from the bioarchaeological record.' *Econ Hum Biol* (Jul 2011); 9(3):284–301. doi: 10.1016/j.ehb.2011.03.004. Epub 2011 Apr 1. PMID: 21507735.

10. Mummert, A., Esche, E., Robinson, J. and Armelagos, G.J., 'Stature and robusticity during the agricultural transition: evidence from the bioarchaeological record.' *Econ Hum Biol* (Jul 2011); 9(3):284–301. doi: 10.1016/j.ehb.2011.03.004. Epub 2011 Apr 1. PMID: 21507735.

11. Barclay, E., 'The Paleo Diet Moves from The Gym to the Doctor's Office.' *npr* (2012). www.npr.org/sections/health-shots/2012/06/02/154166626/the-paleo-diet-moves-from-the-gym-to-the-doctors-office.

12. Cordain, L., Brand-Miller, J., Eaton, S.B., Mann, N., Holt, S. and Speth, J., 'Plant-animal subsistence ratios and macronutrient energy estimations in worldwide hunter-gatherer diets.' *Am J Clin Nutr* 71 (2000); 682–92.

13. Milton, K., 'Reply to L Cordain et al.' *Am J Clin Nutr* 72(2000); 1590–92.

14. Ungar, P., Grine, F. and Teaford, M., 'Diet in Early Homo: A Review of the Evidence and a New Model of Adaptive Versatility.' *Annu. Ev. Anthropol.* 35(2006); 209 228.

15. michaelpollan.com/articles-archive/breaking-ground-the-call-of-the-wild-apple/ Accessed May 5th 2018.

16. Zuk, Marlene, *Paleofantasy: What evolution really tells us about sex, diet, and how we live* (W.W. Norton, 2013), p. 124.

17. www.youtube.com/watch?v=BMOjVYgYaG8&t=2s Tedx, 2013. Debunking the paleo diet.

18. Milton, K., 'Reply to L Cordain *et al.*' *Am J Clin Nutr* 72(2000); 1590–92.

19. McGovern, P.E., Zhang, J., Tang, J., Zhang, Z., Hall, G.R., Moreau ,R.A., Nuñez, A., Butrym, E.D., Richards, M.P., Wang, C.S., Cheng, G., Zhao, Z. and Wang, C., 'Fermented beverages of pre- and proto-historic China.' *Proc Natl Acad Sci U S A* (Dec 21, 2004); 101(51):17593–8. Epub 2004 Dec 8. PMID: 15590771.

20. Kosikowski, F.V., Mistry, V.V., *Cheese and fermented milk foods* Volume 1(1997). Published by F.V. Kosikowski, the University of Wisconsin - Madison Edition 3, illustrated.

21. Rajakumar, K., 'Pellagra in the United States: a historical perspective.' *South Med J.* (Mar 2000); 93(3):272–7. PMID: 10728513.

22. Revedin, A., Aranguren, B., Becattini, R., Longo, L., Marconi, E., Lippi, M., Skakun, N., Sinitsyn, A., Spiridonova, E. and Svoboda, J., 'Thirty thousand-year-old evidence of plant food processing.' *PNAS* 107 (2010); 44; 18815–819.

23. Patin, E. and Quintana-Murci, L., 'Demeter's legacy: rapid changes to our genome imposed by diet.' *Trends Ecol Evol* (Feb 2008); 23(2):56–9. doi: 10.1016/j.tree.2007.11.002. Epub 2008 Jan 11. PMID: 18191277.

24. Reiter, T., Jagoda, E. and Capellini, T.D., 'Dietary Variation and Evolution of Gene Copy Number among Dog Breeds.' *PLoS One* (Feb 10, 2016); 11(2):e0148899. doi: 10.1371/journal.pone.0148899. eCollection 2016. PMID: 26863414.

25. Carrigan, M.A., Uryasev, O., Frye, C.B., Eckman, B.L., Myers, C.R., Hurley, T.D. and Benner, S.A., 'Hominids adapted to metabolize ethanol long before human-directed fermentation.' *Proc Natl Acad Sci U S A* (Jan 13, 2015); 112(2):458–63. doi: 10.1073/pnas.1404167111. Epub 2014 Dec 1. PMID: 25453080.

26. McGovern, PE, et al., 'Fermented beverages of pre- and proto-historic China.' *Proc Natl Acad Sci USA* (Dec 21, 2004); 101(51):17593–8. Epub 2004 Dec 8. PMID: 15590771.

27. http://www.dukandiet.co.uk/the-dukan-diet/4-phases?eprivacy=1 Accessed May 5th 2018.

28. Ibid.

29. Murphy, K.G. and Bloom, S.R., 'Gut hormones and the regulation of energy homeostasis.' *Nature* (Dec 14, 2006); 444(7121):854–9. Review. PMID: 17167473.

30. Tschöp, M., Smiley, D.L. and Heiman, M.L., 'Ghrelin induces adiposity in rodents.' *Nature* (Oct 19, 2000); 407(6806):908–13. PMID: 11057670.

31. Cummings, D.E., Purnell, J.Q., Frayo, R.S., Schmidova, K., Wisse, B.E. and Weigle, D.S., 'A prasprandial rise in plasma ghrelin levels suggests a role in meal initiation in humans.' *Diabetes* (Aug 2001); 50(8):1714–9. PMID: 11473029.

32. Murphy, K.G. and Bloom, S.R., 'Gut hormones . . .'

33. Meek, C.L., Lewis, H.B., Reimann, F., Gribble, F.M., Park, A.J., 'The effect of bariatric surgery on gastrointestinal and pancreatic peptide hormones.' *Peptides* (Mar 2016); 77:28–37. doi: 10.1016/j.peptides.2015.08.013. Epub 2015 Sep 5. Review. PMID: 26344355.

34. Cummings, D.E. and Rubino, F., 'Metabolic surgery for the treatment of type 2 diabetes in obese individuals.' *Diabetologia* (Feb 2018); 61(2):257–64. doi: 10.1007/s00125-017-4513-y. Epub 2017 Dec 9. Review. PMID: 29224190.

35. Manning, S., Pucci, A. and Batterham, R.L. 'Roux-en-Y gastric bypass: effects on feeding behavior and underlying mechanisms.' *J Clin Invest* (Mar 2, 2015); 125(3):939–48. doi: 10.1172/JCI76305. Epub 2015 Mar 2. Review. PMID: 25729850.

36. Chakravartty, .S, Tassinar,i D., Salerno, A., Giorgakis, E. and Rubino, F., 'What is the Mechanism Behind Weight Loss Maintenance with Gastric Bypass?' *Curr Obes Rep* (Jun 2015); 4(2):262–8. doi: 10.1007/s13679-015-0158-7. Review. PMID: 26627220.

37. Simpson, S.J. and Raubenheimer, D., 'Obesity: the protein leverage hypothesis.' *Obes Rev* (May 2005);6(2):133-42. Review. PMID: 15836464.

38. Simpson, S.J., Le Couteur, D.G. and Raubenheimer, D., 'Putting the balance back in diet.' *Cell* (Mar 26, 2015); 161(1):18–23. doi: 10.1016/j.cell.2015.02.033. PMID: 25815981.

39. Ibid.

40. Ibid.

41. Ibid.

42. Ibid.

5. Good gluten, bad gluten and ugly gluten

1. Fasano, A. 'Clinical presentation of celiac disease in the pediatric population.' *Gastroenterology* 128, (2005), S68–73.
2. van Berge-Henegouwen, G. P. and Mulder, C. J., 'Pioneer in the gluten free diet: Willem-Karel Dicke 1905–1962, over 50 years of gluten free diet.' *Gut* 34 (1993), 1473–75.
3. Anderson, C.M., Frazer, A.C., French, J.M., Gerrard, J.W., Sammons, H.G. and Smellie, J.M., 'Cœliac disease: gastro-intestinal studies and the effect of dietary wheat flour.' *Lancet* Volume 259, Issue 6713 (26 April 1952), 836–42.
4. Cooper, B. T., Holmes, G. K., Ferguson, R., Thompson, R. and Cooke, W. T., 'Proceedings: Chronic diarrhoea and gluten sensitivity.' *Gut* 17 (1976), 398.
5. Ellis, A. and Linaker, B. D., 'Non-coeliac gluten sensitivity?' *Lancet* 1 (1978), 1358–59.
6. Sapone, A. et al., 'Differential mucosal IL-17 expression in two gliadin-induced disorders: gluten sensitivity and the autoimmune enteropathy celiac disease.' *Int Arch Allergy Immunol* 152 (2010), 75–80, doi:10.1159/000260087.
7. Davis, W., *Wheat Belly* (Harper Thorsons, UK paperback edition, 2015), Introduction, p. x.
8. 'America the Beautiful' (1910), Lyrics by Katharine Lee Bates, music by Samuel A. Ward.
9. Kasarda, D. D., 'Can an increase in celiac disease be attributed to an increase in the gluten content of wheat as a consequence of wheat breeding?' *J Agric Food Chem* 61 (2013), 1155–59, doi:10.1021/jf305122s.
10. Davis, W., *Wheat Belly*, Introduction p. xii.
11. Shungin, D. et al., 'New genetic loci link adipose and insulin biology to body fat distribution.' *Nature* 518 (2015), 187–96, doi:10.1038/nature14132.
12. Fasano, A. et al., 'Prevalence of celiac disease in at-risk and not-at-risk groups in the United States: a large multicenter study.' *Arch Intern Med* 163 (2003), 286–92.
13. Sapone, A. et al. 'Differential mucosal IL-17 expression in two gliadin-induced disorders: gluten sensitivity and the autoimmune enteropathy celiac disease.' *Int Arch Allergy Immunol* 152 (2010), 75–80, doi:10.1159/000260087.
14. Clemente, M. G. et al., 'Early effects of gliadin on enterocyte intracellular signalling involved in intestinal barrier function.' *Gut* 52 (2003), 218–23.
15. Fasano, A. et al., 'Zonulin, a newly discovered modulator of intestinal permeability, and its expression in coeliac disease.' *Lancet* 355 (2000), 1518–19, doi:10.1016/S0140-6736(00)02169-3; and Wang, W., Uzzau, S., Goldblum, S. E. and Fasano, A., 'Human zonulin, a potential modulator of intestinal tight junctions.' *J Cell Sci* 113 Pt 24 (2000), 4435–40.
16. Sturgeon, C., Lan, J. and Fasano, A., 'Zonulin transgenic mice show altered gut permeability and increased morbidity/mortality in the DSS colitis model.' *Ann N Y Acad Sci* 1397 (2017), 130–42, doi:10.1111/nyas.13343.
17. Gibson, P. R. and Shepherd, S. J., 'Personal view: food for thought – western lifestyle and susceptibility to Crohn's disease. The FODMAP hypothesis.' *Aliment Pharmacol Ther* 21 (2005), 1399–409, doi:10.1111/j.1365-2036.2005.02506.x.
18. Ong, D. K. et al., 'Manipulation of dietary short chain carbohydrates alters the pattern of gas production and genesis of symptoms in irritable bowel syndrome.' *J Gastroenterol Hepatol* 25 (2010), 1366-1373, doi:10.1111/j.1440-1746.2010.06370.x.
19. Staudacher, H. M. and Whelan, K., 'The low FODMAP diet: recent advances

in understanding its mechanisms and efficacy in IBS.' *Gut* 66 (2017), 1517–27, doi:10.1136/gutjnl-2017-313750.

20. Davis, William, *Wheat Belly*, Chapter 5, p. 72.
21. Perlmutter, D., *Grain Brain* (Yellow Kite Books, UK edition, 2014), Introduction, p. 9.
22. Lebwohl, B. *et al.*, 'Long term gluten consumption in adults without celiac disease and risk of coronary heart disease: prospective cohort study.' *BMJ* 357 (2017), j1892, doi:10.1136/bmj.j1892.

6. Blessed are the cheesemakers

1. Gerbault, P. *et al.*, 'Evolution of lactase persistence: an example of human niche construction.' *Philos Trans R Soc Lond B Biol Sci* 366 (2011), 863–77, doi:10.1098/rstb.2010.0268.
2. Boyce, J. A. *et al.*, 'Guidelines for the Diagnosis and Management of Food Allergy in the United States: Summary of the NIAID-Sponsored Expert Panel Report.' *J Allergy Clin Immunol* 126 (2010), 1105–18, doi:10.1016/j.jaci.2010.10.008.
3. Chessa, B. *et al.*, 'Revealing the history of sheep domestication using retrovirus integrations.' *Science* 324 (2009), 532–36, doi:10.1126/science.1170587.
4. Groeneveld, L. F. *et al.*, 'Genetic diversity in farm animals – a review.' *Anim Genet* 41 Suppl 1 (2010), 6–31, doi:10.1111/j.1365-2052.2010.02038.x.
5. Gerbault, P. *et al.*, 'Evolution of lactase persistence . . .'
6. Itan, Y., Powell, A., Beaumont, M. A., Burger, J. and Thomas, M. G., 'The origins of lactase persistence in Europe.' *PLoS Comput Biol* 5 (2009), e1000491, doi:10.1371/journal.pcbi.1000491; and Gerbault, P. et al. Evolution of lactase persistence . . .'
7. Itan, Y., Powell, A., Beaumont, M. A., Burger, J. and Thomas, M. G., 'The origins of lactase persistence . . .'
8. Ibid.
9. Salque, M. *et al.*, 'Earliest evidence for cheesemaking in the sixth millennium BC in northern Europe.' *Nature* 493 (2013), 522–25, doi:10.1038/nature11698.
10. Gerbault, P. *et al.*, 'Evolution of lactase persistence . . .'
11. Ibid.
12. Liu, Y. P. *et al.*, 'Multiple maternal origins of chickens: out of the Asian jungles.' *Mol Phylogenet Evol* 38 (2006), 12–19, doi:10.1016/j.ympev.2005.09.014.
13. Xiang, H. *et al.*, 'Early Holocene chicken domestication in northern China.' *Proc Natl Acad Sci U S A* 111 (2014), 17564–69, doi:10.1073/pnas.1411882111.
14. Giuffra, E. *et al.*, 'The origin of the domestic pig: independent domestication and subsequent introgression.' *Genetics* 154 (2000), 1785–91.
15. Kim, M. Y., Van, K., Kang, Y. J., Kim, K. H. and Lee, S. H., 'Tracing soybean domestication history: From nucleotide to genome.' *Breed Sci* 61 (2012), 445–52, doi:10.1270/jsbbs.61.445.
16. Edenberg, H. J., 'The genetics of alcohol metabolism: role of alcohol dehydrogenase and aldehyde dehydrogenase variants.' *Alcohol Res Health* 30 (2007), 5–13.
17. Exodus 23:19.
18. Guo, J. *et al.*, 'Milk and dairy consumption and risk of cardiovascular diseases and all-cause mortality: dose-response meta-analysis of prospective cohort studies.' *Eur J Epidemiol* 32 (2017), 269–87, doi:10.1007/s10654-017-0243-1; and Tong, X.

et al., 'Cheese Consumption and Risk of All-Cause Mortality: A Meta-Analysis of Prospective Studies.' *Nutrients* 9 (2017), doi:10.3390/nu9010063.

19. Lu, L., Xun, P., Wan, Y., He, K. and Cai, W., 'Long-term association between dairy consumption and risk of childhood obesity: a systematic review and meta-analysis of prospective cohort studies.' *Eur J Clin Nutr* 70 (2016), 414–23, doi:10.1038/ejcn.2015.226.

20. Um, C. Y., Judd, S. E., Flanders, W. D., Fedirko, V. and Bostick, R. M., 'Associations of Calcium and Dairy Products with All-Cause and Cause-Specific Mortality in the Reasons for Geographic and Racial Differences in Stroke (REGARDS) Prospective Cohort Study.' *Nutr Cancer* 69 (2017), 1185-1195, doi:10.1080/01635581.2017.1367946.

7. I am 'plant-based', NOT a vegan

1. Wilson, B., 'Why we fell for clean eating' *Guardian* Long Read, Friday 11th August 2017. www.theguardian.com/lifeandstyle/2017/aug/11/why-we-fell-for-clean-eating

2. Campbell, C. T. and Campbell, T. M., *The China Study* (Benbella Books, Paperback Edition, 2006), Chapter 1, p. 12.

3. Ibid., pp. 12–13.

4. Appleton, B. S. and Campbell, T. C., 'Dietary protein intervention during the post-dosing phase of aflatoxin B1-induced hepatic preneoplastic lesion development.' *J Natl Cancer Inst* 70 (1983), 547–49.

5. Campbell, C. T. and Campbell, T. M., *The China Study*, Chapter 4, p. 71.

6. Ibid., p. 73.

7. Ibid., Introduction, p. 7.

8. Ibid., p. 107.

9. Ibid., Introduction to Part II, 109–10

10. deniseminger.com/the-china-study/ Accessed May 6th, 2018; sciencebasedmed-icine.org/385/ Accessed May 6th, 2018; and www.cholesterol-and-health.com/China-Study.html Accessed May 6th, 2018.

11. O'Connor, T. P., Roebuck, B. D., Peterson, F. and Campbell, T. C., 'Effect of dietary intake of fish oil and fish protein on the development of L-azaserine-induced pre-neoplastic lesions in the rat pancreas.' *J Natl Cancer Inst* 75 (1985), 959–62.

12. Schulsinger, D. A., Root, M. M. and Campbell, T. C., 'Effect of dietary protein quality on development of aflatoxin B1-induced hepatic preneoplastic lesions.' *J Natl Cancer Inst* 81 (1989), 1241–45.

13. Esselstyn Jr., C. B., *Prevent and Reverse Heart Disease: The Revolutionary, Scientifically Proven, Nutrition-Based Cure.* (Avery – Penguin Group First trade paperback edition, 2008).

14. Esselstyn Jr., C. B., Ellis, S. G., Medendorp, S. V. and Crowe, T. D., 'A strategy to arrest and reverse coronary artery disease: a 5-year longitudinal study of a single physician's practice.' *J Fam Pract* 41 (1995), 560–68.

15. Bouvard, V. *et al.* Carcinogenicity of consumption of red and processed meat. *Lancet Oncol* 16 (2015), 1599-1600, doi:10.1016/S1470-2045(15)00444-1.

16. www.cancerresearchuk.org/health-professional/cancer-statistics/risk, Accessed May 6th, 2018.

17. Bouvard, V. *et al.* Carcinogenicity of consumption of red and processed meat. *Lancet Oncol* 16 (2015), 1599-1600, doi:10.1016/S1470-2045(15)00444-1.

18. www.nhs.uk/Livewell/Vegetarianhealth/Pages/Vegetarianhealthqanda.aspx, Accessed May 6th, 2018.

8. Cleanse and detox

1. www.cleanprogram.com/the-program/philosophy Accessed May 6th, 2018.
2. www.juicebaby.co.uk/cleanse/ Accessed May 6th, 2018.
3. rationalwiki.org/wiki/The_dose_makes_the_poison Accessed May 6th, 2018.
4. Isomura, T., Suzuki, S., Origasa, H., Hosono, A., Suzuki, M., Sawada, T., Terao, S., Muto, Y. and Koga, T., 'Liver-related safety assessment of green tea extracts in humans: a systematic review of randomized controlled trials.' *European Journal of Clinical Nutrition* 70 (2016), 1221–29.
5. Edenberg, H. J., 'The genetics of alcohol metabolism: role of alcohol dehydrogenase and aldehyde dehydrogenase variants.' *Alcohol Res Health* 30 (2007), 5–13.
6. Diehl, A. M. and Day, C., 'Cause, Pathogenesis, and Treatment of Nonalcoholic Steatohepatitis.' *N Engl J Med* 377 (2017), 2063–72, doi:10.1056/NEJMra1503519.
7. Jensen, T. et al., 'Fructose and sugar: A major mediator of non-alcoholic fatty liver disease.' *J Hepatol* (2018), doi:10.1016/j.jhep.2018.01.019.

9. The alkalin swindle

1. Young, Robert O. and Young, S. R., *The pH Miracle: Balance your diet, reclaim your health* (Warner Books, Paperback edition, 2003), Chapter 1, p. 6.
2. Ibid, inside cover.
3. Ibid, Chapter 1, p. 4.
4. Ibid, p. 6.
5. Ibid, p. 4.
6. Davis, W. *Wheat Belly* (Harper Thorsons, UK paperback edition, 2015), Chapter 8, p. 116.
7. Campbell, C. T. and Campbell, T. M., *The China Study* Accessed Benbella Books, Paperback Edition, 2006, Chapter 10, p. 205.
8. lady.co.uk/deliciously-healthy-1 Accessed May 6th, 2018.
9. *Clean Eating: The Dirty Truth* BBC *Horizon* (January 19th, 2017), BBC2, Directed by Tristan Quinn. www.bbc.co.uk/programmes/b08bhd29 Accessed May 6th, 2018.
10. www.instagram.com/p/BPdYR6OjdHO/?utm_source=ig_embed Accessed May 6th, 2018.
11. www.amazon.co.uk/Honestly-Healthy-your-body-alkaline/dp/1906417814/ref=s-r_1_1?s=books&ie=UTF8&qid=1525623537&sr=1-1&keywords=honestly+healthy Accessed May 6th, 2018.
12. Corrett, N. and Edgson, V., *Honestly Healthy: Eat with your body in mind, the alkaline way*, (Jacqui Small LLP, Hardback edition, 2012), p. 11.
13. Manchester, K. L., 'Antoine Bechamp: père de la biologie. Oui ou non?' *Endeavour* 25 (2001), 68–73.
14. Ibid.
15. www.phmiracleliving.com/t-cancer-intro.aspx Accessed 6 May 2018.
16. Liberti, M. V. and Locasale, J. W., 'The Warburg Effect: How Does it Benefit Cancer Cells' *Trends Biochem Sci* 41 (2016), 211–18, doi:10.1016/j.tibs.2015.12.001.

17. www.telegraph.co.uk/health-fitness/body/clean-eating-became-dirty-word/ Accessed 6 May 2018.

18. www.sandiegouniontribune.com/sdut-criminal-trial-robert-young-ph-miracle-2016feb03-story.html Accessed 6 May 2018.

19. www.sandiegouniontribune.com/communities/north-county/sd-no-phmiracle-sentence-20170628-story.html Accessed 6 May 2018.

10. Eat like this and look like me

1. Levinovitz, A. *The Gluten Lie, and other myths about what you eat* (Regan Arts, 2015); and www.elle.com/beauty/health-fitness/advice/a28122/detoxing-myth/ (6 May 2018).

2. www.elle.com/uk/life-and-culture/culture/news/a39162/fitness-instagram-women-highest-earner-man/ (6 May 2018).

3. blog.influence.co/instagram-influencers/ (6 May 2018).

4. moonjuice.com/pages/our-story (6 May 2018).

5. Ibid.

6. Ibid.

7. goop.com/wellness/health/the-mysteries-of-the-thyroid/ Accessed 6 May 2018.

8. www.sciencedaily.com/releases/2017/04/170421113306.htm Accessed 6 May 2018.

9. www.theguardian.com/society/2018/feb/12/eating-disorders-nhs-reports-surge-in-hospital-admissions Accessed 6 May, 2018.

10. www.orthorexia.com/ Accessed 6 May, 2018.

11. McGregor, R. *Orthorexia: When healthy eating goes bad* (Watkins, 2017), 25–30.

12. Barnes, M.A. and Caltabiano, M.L., 'The interrelationship between orthorexia nervosa, perfectionism, body image and attachment style.' *Eat Weight Disord* (Mar 2017); 22(1):177–84.

13. www.theguardian.com/lifeandstyle/2015/sep/26/orthorexia-eating-disorder-clean-eating-dsm-miracle-foods Accessed 6 May 2018.

14. Turner, P.G. and Lefevre, C.E., 'Instagram use is linked to increased symptoms of orthorexia nervosa.' *Eat Weight Disord* (June 2017); 22(2):277–84.

15. Ibid.

16. www.bbc.co.uk/news/blogs-ouch-29324937 Accessed 6 May 2018.

17. natashalipman.com/wellness-desperation-chronic-illness/ Accessed 6 May 2018.

18. www.theguardian.com/society/2015/mar/11/belle-gibson-book-publisher-never-verified-cancer-survivor-health-claims Accessed 6 May 2018.

19. https://www.the-pool.com/food-home/food-honestly/2018/2/angry-chef-on-what-we-can-learn-from-belle-gibson-and-the-wellness-community Accessed 6 May 2018.

11. What's the right diet for you?

1. Murphy, K. G. and Bloom, S. R., 'Gut hormones and the regulation of energy homeostasis.' *Nature* 444 (2006), 854–59, doi:10.1038/nature05484.

2. Heshka, S. *et al.*, 'Weight loss with self-help compared with a structured commercial program: a randomized trial.' *JAMA* 289 (2003), 1792–98, doi:10.1001/jama.289.14.1792.

3. Locke, A. E. *et al.*, 'Genetic studies of body mass index yield new insights for obesity biology.' *Nature* 518 (2015), 197–206, doi:10.1038/nature14177.

4. Loos, R. J. and Yeo, G. S., 'The bigger picture of FTO: the first GWAS-identified obesity gene.' *Nat Rev Endocrinol* 10 (2014), 51–61, doi:10.1038/nrendo.2013.227.

5. Gardner, C. D. *et al.*, 'Effect of Low-Fat vs Low-Carbohydrate Diet on 12-Month Weight Loss in Overweight Adults and the Association with Genotype Pattern or Insulin Secretion: The DIETFITS Randomized Clinical Trial.' *JAMA* 319 (2018), 667–79, doi:10.1001/jama.2018.0245.

6. Antoni, R., Johnston, K. L., Collins, A. L. and Robertson, M. D., 'Intermittent v. continuous energy restriction: differential effects on postprandial glucose and lipid metabolism following matched weight loss in overweight/obese participants.' *Br J Nutr* 119 (2018), 507–16, doi:10.1017/S0007114517003890.

7. Estruch, R. *et al.*, 'Primary prevention of cardiovascular disease with a Mediterranean diet.' *N Engl J Med* 368 (2013), 1279–90, doi:10.1056/NEJMoa1200303.

8. Roth, G. A. *et al.*, 'Global and regional patterns in cardiovascular mortality from 1990 to 2013.' *Circulation* 132 (2015), 1667–78, doi:10.1161/CIRCULATIONAHA.114.008720.

9. Wang, D. D. *et al.*, 'Association of Specific Dietary Fats with Total and Cause-Specific Mortality.' *JAMA Intern Med* 176 (2016), 1134–45, doi:10.1001/jamainternmed.2016.2417.

10. Malhotra, A. and O'Neill, D., *The Pioppi Diet: A 21-day Lifestyle Plan*, (Penguin, 2017).

11. www.pioppiprotocol.com/book/ Accessed 7 May 2018.

12. doctoraseem.com/ Accessed 7 May 2018; and letfatbethymedicine.com/ Accessed 7 May 2018.

13. www.penguin.co.uk/articles/find-your-next-read/extracts/2017/jul/the-pioppi-diet-jerk-chicken-recipe/ Accessed 7 May 2018.

14. www.nhlbi.nih.gov/health-topics/dash-eating-plan Accessed 7 May 2018.

15. Juraschek, S. P., Miller, E. R., 3rd, Weaver, C. M. and Appel, L. J., 'Effects of Sodium Reduction and the DASH Diet in Relation to Baseline Blood Pressure.' *J Am Coll Cardiol* 70 (2017), 2841–48, doi:10.1016/j.jacc.2017.10.011.

16. Rai, S. K. et al., 'The Dietary Approaches to Stop Hypertension (DASH) diet, Western diet, and risk of gout in men: prospective cohort study.' *BMJ* 357 (2017), j1794, doi:10.1136/bmj.j1794.

17. Jones, N. R. V., Forouhi, N. G., Khaw, K. T., Wareham, N. J. and Monsivais, P., 'Accordance to the Dietary Approaches to Stop Hypertension diet pattern and cardiovascular disease in a British, population-based cohort.' *Eur J Epidemiol* (2018), doi:10.1007/s10654-017-0354-8.

18. Thaler, R. and Sunstein, C., *Nudge: Improving Decisions about Health, Wealth, and Happiness,* (Yale University Press, 2008), p. 6.

19. www.nobelprize.org/nobel_prizes/economic-sciences/laureates/2017/press.html Accessed 7 May 2018.

20. Hollands, G. J. *et al.*, 'Portion, package or tableware size for changing selection and consumption of food, alcohol and tobacco.' *Cochrane Database Syst Rev* (2015), CD011045, doi:10.1002/14651858.CD011045.pub2.

21. Pechey, R. *et al.*, 'Does wine glass size influence sales for on-site consumption? A multiple treatment reversal design.' *BMC Public Health* 16 (2016), 390, doi:10.1186/s12889-016-3068-z.

22. Swift, D. L., Johannsen, N. M., Lavie, C. J., Earnest, C. P. and Church, T. S., 'The role of exercise and physical activity in weight loss and maintenance.' *Prog Cardiovasc Dis* 56 (2014), 441–47, doi:10.1016/j.pcad.2013.09.012.

23. Finlayson, G., Bryant, E., Blundell, J. E. and King, N. A., 'Acute compensatory eating following exercise is associated with implicit hedonic wanting for food.' *Physiol Behav* 97 (2009), 62–67, doi:10.1016/j.physbeh.2009.02.002.

24. www.telegraph.co.uk/sport/olympics/2563451/Michael-Phelps-the-extraordinary-12000-calorie-diet-that-fuels-greatest-ever-Olympian-Beijing-Olympics-2008.html Accessed 7 May 2018.

25. Finlayson, G., Bryant, E., Blundell, J. E. and King, N. A., 'Acute compensatory eating . . .'

26. Jakicic, J. M., Rogers, R. J., Davis, K. K. and Collins, K. A., 'Role of Physical Activity and Exercise in Treating Patients with Overweight and Obesity.' *Clin Chem* 64 (2018), 99–107, doi:10.1373/clinchem.2017.272443; and Finlayson, G., Bryant, E., Blundell, J. E. and King, N. A., 'Acute compensatory eating . . .'

27. King, N. A., Hopkins, M., Caudwell, P., Stubbs, R. J. and Blundell, J. E., 'Beneficial effects of exercise: shifting the focus from body weight to other markers of health.' *Br J Sports Med* 43 (2009), 924–27, doi:10.1136/bjsm.2009.065557.

12. The perfect diet written in your genes

1. www.dnafit.com/ Accessed 7 May 2018; and https://www.nutrigenomix.com/ Accessed 7 May 2018.

2. Edenberg, H. J., 'The genetics of alcohol metabolism: role of alcohol dehydrogenase and aldehyde dehydrogenase variants.' *Alcohol Res Health* 30 (2007), 5–13.

3. Itan, Y., Powell, A., Beaumont, M. A., Burger, J. and Thomas, M. G., 'The origins of lactase persistence in Europe.' *PLoS Comput Biol* 5 (2009), e1000491, doi:10.1371/journal.pcbi.1000491.

4. Montague, C. T. *et al.*, 'Congenital leptin deficiency is associated with severe early-onset obesity in humans.' *Nature* 387 (1997), 903–08, doi:10.1038/43185.

5. Locke, A. E. *et al.*, 'Genetic studies of body mass index yield new insights for obesity biology.' *Nature* 518 (2015), 197–206, doi:10.1038/nature14177.

6. Ibid.

7. Montague, C. T. *et al.*, 'Congenital leptin deficiency is associated with severe early-onset obesity in humans.' *Nature* 387 (1997), 903–08, doi:10.1038/43185.

8. Practice Committee of American Society for Reproductive Medicine in collaboration with Society for Reproductive, E. and Infertility, 'Optimizing natural fertility: a committee opinion.' *Fertil Steril* 100 (2013), 631–37, doi:10.1016/j.fertnstert.2013.07.011.

9. van der Klaauw, A. A. *et al.*, 'Divergent effects of central melanocortin signalling on fat and sucrose preference in humans.' *Nat Commun* 7 (2016), 13055, doi:10.1038/ncomms13055.

10. Jakicic, J. M. *et al.*, 'Effect of Wearable Technology Combined With a Lifestyle Intervention on Long-term Weight Loss: The IDEA Randomized Clinical Trial.' *JAMA* 316 (2016), 1161–71, doi:10.1001/jama.2016.12858.

11. Locke, A. E. *et al.*, 'Genetic studies of body mass index yield new insights for obesity biology.' *Nature* 518 (2015), 197–206, doi:10.1038/nature14177; and Loos, R. J.,

'Genetic determinants of common obesity and their value in prediction.' *Best Pract Res Clin Endocrinol Metab* 26 (2012), 211-226, doi:10.1016/j.beem.2011.11.003.

12. Cong, L. *et al.*, 'Multiplex genome engineering using CRISPR/Cas systems.' *Science* 339 (2013), 819–23, doi:10.1126/science.1231143; Jinek, M. et al., 'A programmable dual-RNA-guided DNA endonuclease in adaptive bacterial immunity.' *Science* 337 (2012), 816–21, doi:10.1126/science.1225829; and Mali, P. et al., 'RNA-guided human genome engineering via Cas9.' *Science* 339 (2013), 823–26, doi:10.1126/science.1232033.

INDEX